THE
HEART
AND ITS HEALING PLANTS

"Until recently Western science saw the heart as a very sophisticated pump. Over the past 30 years research has shown the heart is much more, with significant endocrine and nervous system function. Ancient cultures perceived that the heart was the source of life, emotions, bravery, the self, and spirit. Wolf D. Storl's *The Heart and Its Healing Plants* is a unique book that bridges cultures, centuries, myth, and science to expand our knowledge of the heart and the plants that can be used to heal broken hearts literally, figuratively, and ceremonially as well."

DAVID WINSTON, RH(AHG), AUTHOR OF *ADAPTOGENS: HERBS FOR STRENGTH, STAMINA, AND STRESS RELIEF*

"What happens when we cross one of the most original, deep-thinking, spiritual minds of the era with one of the most complicated, least understood, important organs in the body? We get an amazing book by Wolf D. Storl on the heart, holism medicine, and herbalism. But *amazing* is too limiting a word. What we have here is a *foundation* for all future holistic work on these subjects. We want to know the deep, ancient, indigenous stories of the plants as well as the most modern pharmacology. We want to plumb the depths of the human heart in its every facet. That's what we have here."

MATTHEW WOOD, AUTHOR OF *HOLISTIC MEDICINE AND THE EXTRACELLULAR MATRIX*

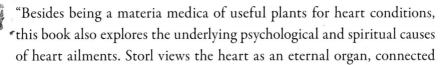

"Besides being a materia medica of useful plants for heart conditions, this book also explores the underlying psychological and spiritual causes of heart ailments. Storl views the heart as an eternal organ, connected to the universe and the divine. He calls for a return to nature's own biorhythm and to the pulses of life and joy that can be found by reconnecting to the natural world. By paying attention to dreams, the cycles of the seasons, and to the sun and moon, we can heal the heart of our being and find calm, love, and peace in the eye of life's storm. This is a valuable book that will help us to navigate our stressed, fast-paced, and mechanized modern lifestyle."

ELLEN EVERT HOPMAN, AUTHOR OF *SECRET MEDICINES FROM YOUR GARDEN*, *A DRUID'S HERBAL FOR THE SACRED EARTH YEAR*, AND *THE SACRED HERBS OF YULE AND CHRISTMAS*

"A masterful synthesis of spirituality and science that is relevant to everyone who has a heart. Storl traces herbalism from its deep roots in the European herbal tradition and the vision of Hildegard to the modern use of cardioactive plants and their chemistry in cardiology. Now we need the same quality and depth of scholarship applied to all our organs!"

DAVID HOFFMANN, FNIMH, RH, AUTHOR OF *MEDICAL HERBALISM* AND *THE HERBAL HANDBOOK*

"*The Heart and Its Healing Plants* gets to the core of heart health by addressing the history, folklore, spirit, science, and emotional factors that affect the cardiovascular system. It weaves a fascinating look at the deepest aspects of healing the heart from many world cultures over a span of centuries."

BRIGITTE MARS, AHG, AUTHOR OF *THE SEXUAL HERBAL*, *ADDICTION-FREE NATURALLY*, AND *NATURAL REMEDIES FOR MENTAL AND EMOTIONAL HEALTH*

"Wolf D. Storl presents a holistic view of common heart illnesses. He does not only deal with their physical causes but also tackles the harmful psychic attitudes and misdirected life goals that enable diseases. This is a great book to understand, prevent, and cure heart disease."

CHRISTOPHER VASEY, N.D., AUTHOR OF *NATURAL ANTIBIOTICS AND ANTIVIRALS* AND *THE ACID-ALKALINE DIET FOR OPTIMUM HEALTH*

THE
HEART
AND ITS HEALING PLANTS

Traditional Herbal Remedies
and Modern Heart Conditions

Wolf D. Storl, Ph.D.

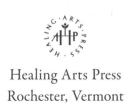

Translated by Christine Storl

Healing Arts Press

Rochester, Vermont

Healing Arts Press
One Park Street
Rochester, Vermont 05767
www.HealingArtsPress.com

Healing Arts Press is a division of Inner Traditions International

Originally published in German in 2009 under the title *Das Herz: Und seine heilenden Pflanzen* by AT Verlag
First U.S. edition published in 2024 by Healing Arts Press

Note to the reader: This book is intended as an informational guide. The information has been presented to the best of the author's knowledge and has been reviewed with the utmost care. The remedies, approaches, and techniques described herein are meant to supplement, and not to be a substitute for, professional medical care or treatment. They should not be used to treat a serious ailment without prior consultation with a qualified health care professional.

Cataloging-in-Publication Data for this title is available from the Library of Congress

ISBN 978-1-64411-838-2 (print)
ISBN 978-1-64411-839-9 (ebook)

Printed and bound in in China by Reliance Printing Co., Ltd

10 9 8 7 6 5 4 3 2 1

Text design and layout by Virginia Scott Bowman
This book was typeset in Garamond Premier Pro and Gill Sans with Cinzel and Gill Sans used as display typefaces

To send correspondence to the author of this book, mail a first-class letter to the author c/o Inner Traditions • Bear & Company, One Park Street, Rochester, VT 05767, and we will forward the communication, or contact the author directly at **storl.de/english-books-by-wolf-d-storl**.

Thanks to my loyal readers and the masters
of herbalism who showed me the way.

Special thanks to Marianne Ruoff, M.D., and
Elke Mohaupt, M.D., who took the time to read the book and
send me valuable suggestions for
corrections and changes based on their wealth of
medical knowledge and experience.

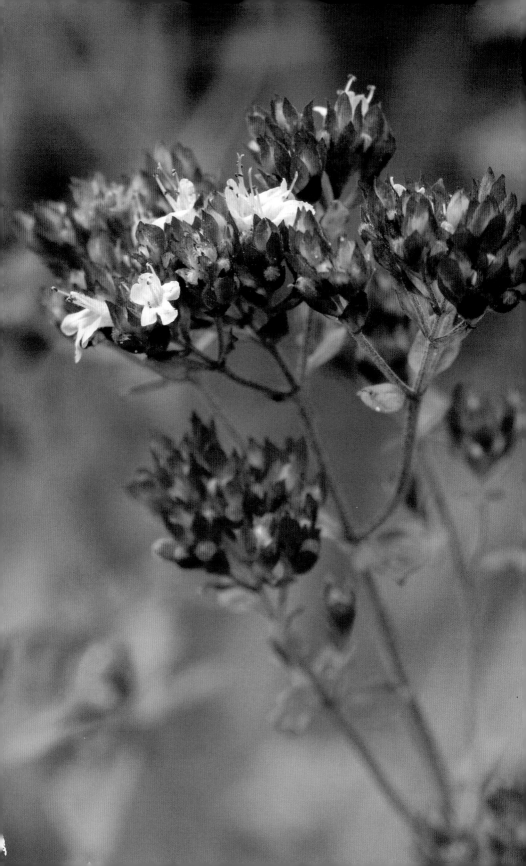

CONTENTS

PREFACE

To really know something—not simply believe or think,
but to know—is only possible with the whole heart.

REINHARD FRIEDL, CARDIAC SURGEON

MOST CARDIOLOGISTS VIEW THE HEART AS A PUMP—a highly
complicated one, but nevertheless only a mechanical pump that, in the
event of a malfunction, doctors try to repair with the help of comprehensive high-tech medicine and synthetic pharmaceuticals. Medicinal
herbs rarely play a role in any of this. Elke Mohaupt, M.D., a specialist
in internal medicine, wrote to me in a personal letter:

> The fact is that the knowledge of the effects of healing plants in
> our medicine—especially in cardiology—has not (yet?) been prop-
> erly addressed. That is a shame because it is such an exciting field,
> especially for us doctors! I recommend herbal supplements—thank
> goodness they still exist—for nervous heart problems and there is a
> good success rate. Many of my colleagues (and particularly the car-
> diologists!) are unaware of these preparations. I also think a reason
> for the increasing deterioration of phytotherapeutic knowledge in
> the medical profession is the fact that all herbal medicines must be
> paid for by the patients themselves, and are not covered by ordinary
> health insurance. This has the following consequences: (1) there are
> practically no pharmaceutical representatives who discuss herbal

medicines, which would encourage our interest in phytotherapy; and (2) there is less appreciation for plant medicine on the part of the patients themselves. Herbal medication is not based on an "official prescription" that has value because you get something—free, or at least seemingly free—when you hand it over to the pharmacist, but instead it is only a recommendation that is not covered by medical insurance, so you must pay out of pocket for it. Plant medicines are also ignored when it comes to medical research; they are seen as an aspect of medical history that has long been superseded.

As far as the "pump" is concerned, there is even a recent, rather reluctant reassessment among the most forward-thinking of cardiologists: the heart cannot be explained in mechanistic terms alone. This organ, which gives us the rhythm of life, is there at the beginning of our existence. It is the first fully developed organ; it starts to beat three weeks after conception and is completely formed seven weeks after fertilization. The development of the cerebral cortex only begins in the eighth week, when the heart has already been in operation for some time. In other words, the functional heart, which can transport blood and nutrients, is a prerequisite for the development of the brain and all the other organs.

Researchers at the University of Montreal found that when undifferentiated embryonic stem cells are sprinkled with the love hormone oxytocin, something magical happens: they connect, transform into heart muscle cells, and start to beat synchronously (Friedl 2019, 132). The love hormone thus triggers the first of the heartbeats that will accompany us for a lifetime.

In the human organism, oxytocin is generated not only in the brain but also in the heart. And it is not just the brain, but the heart, too, which releases the hormone during a loving gaze, a hug, or during lovemaking and its climax. This biochemical messenger enables a deep heart-to-heart connection. Oxytocin has a cardioprotective effect: it lowers blood pressure, calms the pulse, and lowers cortisone levels—it makes the heart happy. Moreover, it also inhibits the release of inflammatory mediators, thus blocking the development of arteriosclerosis. The heart of the fetus produces more oxytocin than the heart of an adult. Just before birth, it releases even more of this love hormone, which prepares the mother's organism for the birth and ultimately initiates labor. After birth, the hormone helps the uterus involute; it also stimulates the mammary glands and promotes milk flow. During breastfeeding and when a mother and her infant are in direct physical contact, their hearts begin to beat in sync.

The heart and the brain are not separated. It is now known that they communicate with one another via the autonomous nervous system, via breathing, and so on. The brain pulsates with the same rhythm of the heartbeat; craniosacral therapy is based on this knowledge. The ancient Greeks knew ten types of pulse; in Chinese medicine, twenty-eight different subtle oscillations (pulses) can be felt. Complex scientific experiments were able to detect signals in the brain that came from the heart. The brain responds to these signals that affect our perception and decisions. According to the latest research results, the traditional belief that the heart has something to do with compassion and courage no longer seems so improbable (Friedl 2019, 191). The heart has cardio-cognitive consciousness—it senses when something is coherent; it reacts to emotions.

The synchronization of heartbeats is not only restricted to mothers and their infants. A synchronous harmony of hearts also arises in other situations—for example, when people sing together in a choir, engage in group mantra singing, or conduct rituals and pujas. The same phenomenon occurs for groups of people involved in risky or dangerous situations, such as with medical teams during difficult operations or soldiers during a confrontation in battle.

Even on a biological level, the heart is indeed the organ of love and compassion, in which—as the mystics say—our divine Self resides. In antiquity, in alchemy, in the astrological plantlore of the Renaissance, and in the ancient philosophy of India the sun in the heavens was regarded as the heart of the macrocosm. The green, photosynthetic vegetation also develops and lives in harmony with the sun; it is directly connected to this cosmic pulse-generator. Therefore, plants can help us to find our own rhythm of life—and to regain it if we have lost it. In the following pages, we will take a closer look at some of the plants that are especially suited for this.

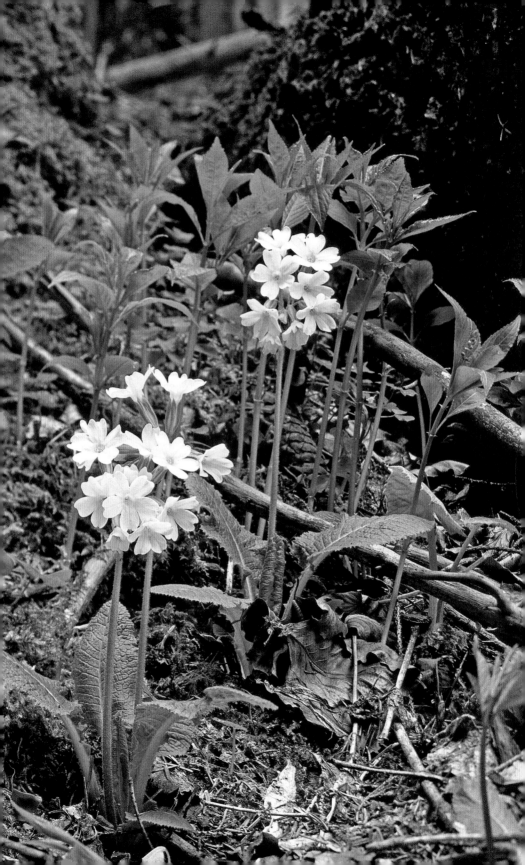

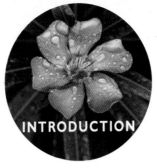

THE HEART OF THE MATTER

GIVEN THE CRISES TODAY of the technologized Western world, in which the human heart is constantly trying to keep up with a fast, usually machine-driven pace, it is not surprising that heart ailments are essentially the number one killer—indeed, they are second only to iatrogenic deaths (those that result from the activity of doctors or surgeons).* After heart ailments, the next two major causes of death are cancer and strokes.

Coronary heart diseases have become a big business. It seems obvious that the human heart is barely able to take the conditions that

---

*"Yes, my dear colleagues, we know what the major cause of death is in the world today," announced one of the doctors during his lecture at the ethno-medical congress that took place at the Ludwig Maximilian University of Munich in October 2007. The audience assumed the answer was obvious: coronary diseases and cancer. The lecturer continued: "We doctors are the main cause of death." Indeed, the facts speak for themselves. According to the *Journal of the American Medical Association,* 106,000 patients die each year due to the side effects of properly prescribed medication, while 2,216,000 patients experience serious chronic damage. The study does not even list statistics for false diagnoses, mistakes in dosage, and the misuse of medication (Lazarou et al. 1998, 1200). A research study led by Dr. Jürgen Fröhlich, director of the Department of Clinical Pharmacology at the Medical University in Hannover, Germany, calculated that in German hospitals alone the internists recorded 58,000 patients yearly as having died due to the side effects of medication (Schnurrer and Fröhlich 2003). On top of all of this there are the mistakes made in treatment, the hospital-spawned infections, and other causes, which are responsible for hundreds of thousands of fatalities per year. Dr. Vernon Coleman comments: "Not even members of the medical establishment can deny that doctors are one of the main causes of sickness and death—to a greater extent than all accidents combined and on par with cancer and coronary diseases" (2006, 30).

prevail in our modern world of machines and technology: stress and anxiety, job insecurity, pent-up anger, and lovelessness. Then there is the constant stream of terrible news on television—wars that involve us indirectly or even personally; globalized criminal networks involving things such as child pornography; young people dying from deadly drugs such as fentanyl; or the recent increase of myocarditis apparently resulting from Covid vaccinations, for instance—and the insecure feeling of having very little say in one's own life while living under an increasing amount of government regulations. All of these things and many more take a toll on the human heart that is generally underestimated. They represent a societal-cultural problem that requires a remedy, for it also filters down and directly affects our health. Many of today's bright minds have convincingly questioned the belief that a body is basically just a machine that needs maintenance or repair when the parts wear out. It has become more and more apparent that disease has a psychosomatic aspect and that our emotions have a very real effect on our health. In the realm of heart disease, this seems to be even more the case than with other diseases. The stress of living in a modern industrial society makes it difficult to experience great joy of life—joy that has traditionally always been perceived as experience of the heart.

In this book, we will examine from the perspective of ethnobotany and cultural anthropology how old European cultures (my area of expertise) related to the heart and also touch on the views of some other indigenous peoples. We will consider various worldviews regarding the subject. How were heart diseases defined? What methods of healing were used? Why and how were they applied in treatment? Such information should not be considered as a medical guidebook. While the topic of modern medicine will not be ignored in these pages, it is not my main area of interest. It is also not my intention to preach to or discredit medical professionals with this entirely different point of view, nor do I wish to meddle in modern cardiology by suggesting which plants to use for high blood pressure, arrhythmia, angina pectoris, or heart failure. Numerous books of this sort are available. My main emphasis is on broadening our horizons with respect to how we define the heart—through ethnobotanical and ethnomedicinal explorations, we can expand our view regarding heart problems and learn about the plants that have an age-old connection to the heart. The plants will also be presented more as spiritual allies of the heart than as vehicles for active ingredients that help various heart disorders; although these aspects are not neglected here either, they are, however, not my main concern.

Often when one has burned all their bridges and stands on the threshold of a new phase in life, prophetic dreams may come to help guide the way. This was the case for me when, at age forty-four, I returned to the land of my birth and my ancestors, which I had left when I was eleven years old. After some twenty-five years spent in the United States and two years in India—which revealed itself to me as a veritable "country of the gods"—my wife and I ended up living in the moors of East Frisia in northern Germany, where I still have some relatives. It was not completely clear what I would be doing professionally, except that I planned to continue writing books as I had been doing for some years. Our savings were running low, and the future was still a mystery. I dreamed of two houses that we could live in: the first was a brightly lit modern house, Bauhaus-style, made of glass and artificial materials and full of appliances; the second was a large rustic house in the woods, with a warm fire blazing in the hearth—and not much electric light. A higher being, an angel or a god—was it Wotan?—was showing me that I could choose which house I preferred, and this would then become our dwelling place. I chose the house with the fire—I intuitively sensed that the hearth in the middle of the house had emanated a warm invitation to my own heart.

I ended up choosing the path of the heart. For the divine Self lives in the heart and will not be found on the path of external appearances. If the latter path is chosen, one will invariably be reminded at some later point that it is necessary to return to the heart. The fast pace of modern life usually takes its toll, and the heart becomes hardened, or painful, or loses its rhythm. It may even break down. The art of healing the heart—and the plants that help this to happen—is the subject of this book. For these plants must indeed know about this kind of healing, because they live day and night with the cosmic rhythm of the cosmic heart, the sun.

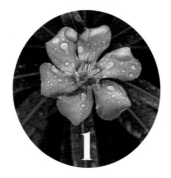

THE HEART—JUST A PUMP?

The medical art is rooted in the heart.

If your heart is false, then the physician inside you is
also false.

If it is righteous, then the physician is also righteous.

PARACELSUS (1530)

THE HEART, ACCORDING TO A MODERN MEDICAL dictionary, is the muscular central organ of the circulatory system; in an adult, the hollow organ made of muscular tissue, and weighing approximately 10.5 ounces, functions as a double-acting pump (Minker 1992, 124). This small high-performance motor, this "580-horsepower machine"—as Austrian heart surgeon Dr. Ferdinand Waldenberger calls it—pumps blood out of the cavities sixty to eighty times a minute. The corresponding circulatory system stretches over some 62,130 miles, or two-and-a-half times around the entire Earth. The heart beats about 100,000 times a day, more than four million times a year, and around three billion times in a normal lifetime. Four to seven quarts of blood flow per minute, or 2,000 gallons per day. During a normal lifetime, the human heart pumps enough blood to fill two oil tankers (Waldenberger 2003, 15).

From a modern perspective, this impressive pump system proves to be frail enough:

- The muscle can weaken (cardiac insufficiency).
- The valves, which close the atria and the veins so that no blood flows backward, can fail (cardiac valve insufficiency).
- The tubes can calcify, clog, and become constricted (arteriosclerosis).
- A blood clot (thrombus) can completely block an artery, causing a heart attack and ending in sudden death. Another term for this is an acute myocardial infarction.*

All sorts of things can, of course, go wrong with this little machine. Fortunately, we have a veritable heart industry—full of highly qualified health engineers and "mechanics"—that can keep the pump going. State-of-the-art diagnostic methods, such as the electrocardiogram (ECG or EKG) and, depending on the symptoms, a cardiac stress test, provide a factual diagnosis. Coronary angiocardiography, cardiac catheter examination, and/or an ultrasound examination (echocardiography) may follow. Other procedures ensure repair, good maintenance, and the optimal functioning of the stressed body machine. Magnetic resonance imaging (MRI) and computer tomography (CT) may also be used before a transplant or for clarifying rare problems. Here are a few interventions:

- For cardiomyopathy (disease of the heart muscle) and dangerously high blood pressure there are beta-blockers, calcium antagonists, and ACE inhibitors, which lower the blood pressure. There are so-called antiarrhythmic drugs for alleviating disturbances in heart rhythm. Even better for tired hearts is the cardiac pacemaker, an implanted electrical device that generates pulses which stimulate a regulated heartbeat. There are also heart medications derived from plants, such as foxglove (*digitalis*), lily of the valley (*convallaria*),

---

Infarction (from Latin *infarctus,* "stuffed into, filled") was a medical term used to describe an intestinal blockage in the eighteenth century. In the nineteenth century it was used to describe blood congestion, and in the twentieth century it came to describe the dying of heart tissue due to clogged vessels.

hellebore (*helleborus*), genista (*genista; cytisus*), climbing oleander (*Strophanthus gratus*), or laurel rose (*Nerum oleander*). Many of them contain positive inotropic cardiac glycosides, which are so poisonous they basically scare the body into making the heart pump stronger to rid itself of the toxins via the liver and kidneys.* These cardiac glycosides are now produced synthetically and are a billion-dollar-a-year business.

◆ Specialists can replace problematic valves with an artificial valvular prosthesis or a bio prosthesis, such as from a donor heart or a pig's heart.

◆ In the case of vasoconstriction, operative measures are also taken in the form of a bypass—for example, like alleviating a traffic jam by rerouting the traffic, the constricted section of the coronary blood vessel is bypassed by using a vein from the leg or arm. In the United States approximately 300,000 patients a year undergo a bypass operation. Moreover, there is also percutaneous transluminal coronary angioplasty (PTCA), in which a tiny rubber hose is placed into the coronary blood vessel and then inflated to widen the constricted vessel. Commonly called stents, small tubes made of metal or artificial material are also placed in the blood vessels. In modern Western countries, this expensive procedure is carried out on an average of 250,000 people per population of 80 million each year.

◆ In the case of patients with end-stage heart failure who remain symptomatic despite optimal medical therapy, the heart itself can be surgically removed and a donor heart transplanted in its place, similarly to how a worn-out car engine can be replaced with a new one.

These treatments all sound well and good and give the impression that the experts have everything well under control. Nevertheless, there are more than a few issues that arise. Even though they are effective, many heart medicines have undesirable side effects. Beta-blockers, for example, can constrict the blood vessels and cause sleeping disorders and

---

*Positive inotropic agents influence the heart muscle's beating strength and its ability to contract.

impotence. Antiarrhythmics can cause tinnitus, impaired vision, sensitivity to sunlight, and even weaken the heart muscle (Maxen, Hoffbauer, and Heeke 2005, 343). The most dangerous side effect of antiarrhythmics, which include beta-blockers, is irregular heartbeat—meaning they can cause the very symptoms that they should be alleviating.

Pacemakers are not as sensitive to electromagnetic fields (such as those generated by microwave ovens, for example) as they were at first. However, there are still warnings that caution should be exercised near very strong electromagnetic fields and when carrying cell phones; a cell phone should be kept at a distance of about twelve inches from the pacemaker, which is usually implanted under the right collarbone.

Artificial heart valves last for a few years at most, and they result in numerous red blood cells being crushed each time they close. They also provide ideal conditions for blood clots, which is not the case with natural heart valves. If a mechanical prosthesis is used as a heart valve, the recipient must regularly take medication (blood thinners) that has severe side effects; she or he remains a permanent patient.

A bypass operation can cost anywhere from 50,000 to 100,000 dollars. It doesn't take a mathematical genius to recognize that this is another huge, billion-dollar business (Chopra 2001, 19). In industrialized countries, 70,000 such surgical interventions per population of 80 million occur yearly. The cost-benefit ratio is dismal when one considers that for 10 to 15% of the patients, the valve fails after only one year. Studies have also shown that these expensive operative practices are barely capable of significantly extending a patient's life (Blech 2005, 179). The American doctor Harvey Bigelsen wonders whether the sense of feeling better after a bypass operation might not actually be a result of the nerves that register pain having been cut (Bigelsen 2011, 70).

Despite the billions that are spent to keep the pump-and-tube system functioning smoothly, coronary diseases remain number one among the deadly diseases in the modern world. Approximately half of the deaths in industrialized Western societies can be chalked up to coronary disease. In 1996, the German medical journal *Ärztezeitung* cited approximately one million heart attacks per year in Germany alone, with 200,000 of them resulting in death. In the United states in 1997, nearly one million people died of coronary diseases (Schmertzing 2002, 72). In addition, some 600,000 new patients in Germany develop coronary disorders each year—a typical statistic for a modern Western country.

HEART REMEDIES OF INDIGENOUS PEOPLES

With regard to heart health problems, things have not always been like they are now—neither for our ancestors nor for any traditional and indigenous peoples. In either case, heart ailments were hardly known. Of course, the heart pounds wildly in the face of danger, or becomes pain-ridden through suffering and sorrow, or stands still in extreme shock, or can even be broken. A heart might also be stolen, charmed, or bewitched. But heart diseases as we know them in the modern, industrialized age were—and still are in so-called developing countries—essentially unknown. When ethnopharmacologists search through the healing lore of indigenous peoples, they find very little that pertains to any kinds of heart ailments.

Indigenous peoples—hunter-gatherers as well as hoe-farmers—have always made use of a wide range of healing herbs, barks, and roots. These medicinal plants reflect the health problems of the people. Many of these cures involve hemostatic plants, which are used to stop bleeding, heal wounds, and fight topical infections. There are also numerous healing plants for gastrointestinal illnesses, stomach cramps, diarrhea, worms, and skin rashes; and many purgatives are found that induce vomiting, diarrhea, sweating, or urination—bodily reactions that help rid oneself of toxins, including such afflictions as "magic arrows," "worms," and "evil spirits."

In colder northern climates, indigenous peoples made use of various plants for the lungs, such as colt's foot, angelica, witch hazel, heath milkwort, burnet, and thyme. Lung problems were fairly common due to the cold climate and the smoke from the open fires in the houses. Healing plants containing salacin—such as willow bark or meadowsweet—helped with rheumatism and arthritis, which were common ailments in places where people slept on cold, damp earthen floors. Painkillers, diuretics, anti-inflammatory agents, and plants for healing broken bones were also found in abundance among European indigenous peoples. In addition, a profound knowledge regarding consciousness-altering natural drugs, which were used in a sacral-cultural context (and mainly by the men), was, and is, present. The women possessed a wide spectrum of gynecological healing plants for menstrual difficulties and various female disorders, as well as plants that supported fertility and birth (Lipp 1996, 21; Wolters 1999, 79). There were also plenty of plants used by women to bewitch men. But cardiac medicines are hardly found in indigenous herbal lore. If one does come across a cardiac medicine, it will most likely be a plant with glycosides, which strongly affect the heart and can be used to poison the tips of arrows. For instance, the Celts applied the poisonous juice of hellebore to the tips of the spears and arrows used for hunting deer. The African Pygmies made a decoction of the seeds and roots of plants containing strophanthin (such as the aforementioned climbing oleander or laurel rose) and soaked their arrow tips in it for hunting elephants. No matter where the animal was hit with the arrow, it would die of catalepsy and heart failure. In modern cardiac medicine, strophanthin is regarded as a kind of wonder drug; in very exact and controlled doses, it is administered as an injection for acute heart insufficiency (bradycardia) and cardiac decompensation.

I became quite aware how native people did not have a tradition with cardiac medicine when I was undertaking ethnobotanical excursions in the Bighorn Mountains in Wyoming and Montana with my Cheyenne friend Bill Tallbull. The Cheyenne had been forced onto a small reservation. They had to endure the authorities making harsh demands on them, religious fanatics trying to convert them, teachers punishing them for speaking their own language, social workers snooping into their family matters, and do-gooders questioning the old Cheyenne ways and values, all of which was especially confusing for the younger generation. And then there was the daily struggle to survive amid a lack of employment opportunities and the unscrupulous actions of the big mining corporations that disregarded traditional land-use rights and moved in with loud machinery, scraping away the sacred soil. The culture of these once-proud bison hunters was further threatened by hopelessness, violence, alcoholism, social disintegration, and the loss of their native tongue. The old medicine man had taken all this so much to heart that his heart was in pain.

"But you native Americans have so many healing plants," I said. "Don't you have healing plants for heart ailments?"

"Before we were forced on to a reservation and we took on the life-style and eating habits of white people, we had no heart ailments," he answered. "Diabetes was also unknown, which is now a big problem for our people. We had no tooth decay, cancer, or extreme obesity. Those diseases were unknown to us, so we have no healing plants for them. We drink *Mo e'-emohk' shin* [Elk mint]* as a tea when we have intense pain in the chest due to coughing or if someone has a weak, dispirited heart. We pray for help, but sometimes it takes a long time before the plant spirits take pity on us and show us their healing powers."

HEART AILMENTS IN OLD EUROPEAN TRADITIONS OF FOLK MEDICINE

For the various old European cultures—whether in the Mediterranean regions or in the northern woodlands of the Slavic, Germanic, and Celtic peoples—heart disease was as little known as it was among Native Americans. The heart was perceived as the place where vitality and courage originated; it was never understood as a mechanical pump. Its rhythmic heartbeat was the very pulse of life—just like how in nature the cycles of day and night, or the ocean tides, represent life's natural rhythm. According to older Germanic traditions, a heart was either big or small: a coward had a small heart, whereas a courageous person had a big one. The heart was seen as either warm or cold, hard

---

*Blue Giant Hyssop, *Agastache anethiodora* or *A. foeniculum*.

or soft; if someone was greedy, haughty, arrogant, or merciless, this was associated with a cold and hard heart. By contrast, a good person had a soft and warm heart, capable of sympathy, kindness, and compassion. Heart ailments were therefore seen as sicknesses of the soul and not as organic or functional maladies.

In the old folk medicine that had its roots in earlier Celtic, Germanic, and Slavic traditions, heart ailments were seen as having supernatural causes. When the chest and the diaphragm were in actual physical pain—such as with what we call "heartburn," gastric discomfort or nausea (which the French call *mal au cœur,* literally "heart sickness"), or pleurisy—this was also attributed to the heart.* If the heart was beating violently, or experiencing cramps or stabbing pain, it was believed that "nagging" or "pissing" "worms" were the culprit, or other invisible disease-causing evil spirits and demons, or perhaps malicious elves. Witchcraft or sorcery might also be the source of the problem. Here we will consider a few of the common diagnoses from quite old traditions of European folk medicine.

A Heart Full of Straw

When someone's heart became increasingly weak, to the point that the person had practically lost all strength and zest to live, it was assumed that a witch or sorceress was tampering with the victim's heart at night while he or she was sleeping.† It was imagined that such entities sometimes "cut the heart out and ate it, then stuffed straw or wood into the chest cavity" (Bächtold-Stäubli 1987, III:1811; Grimm 2003, 875). The following question is cited in a penitential and confessional book belonging to Bishop

---

*These gastro-cardiac ailments correlate to the now somewhat outdated Roemheld syndrome.

†A "witch" in this context has nothing to do with the emancipated, enlightened female figures that are presented in the contemporary women's movement. They were also not necessarily the herbal healing women, heathen priestesses, or midwives who had been condemned by the church. Wicked witches were believed to be invisible astral entities that were sent out by evil beings to harm others. Due to their shamanic ability to go into a trance, these kinds of witches could enter the body of a cat or a night bird, or could hide "between the bark and the tree."

Burchard of Worms (died 1025) and is one example among many that reflects the disdain the church held toward the older, traditional beliefs. It is to be used for interrogating a suspected witch.

> Do you believe what many women believe and hold true, women who have reverted to Satan? Namely that in the silence of restless nights, although you lie in bed and your man is asleep at your bosom while you are physically behind closed doors, you are able to depart and cross the spaces of the world with others laboring in the same deluded state, and with invisible weapons slay baptized Christians who are redeemed through the blood of Christ, boil their flesh and consume it, and stuff straw or wood or other things in the place where their heart was, and reanimate those you have eaten and extend their lease on life.

This is an archaic belief, which can also be found among the North Germanic peoples—for example, in the *Laxdœla Saga* from Iceland (Hasenfratz 2011, 87).

A Worm in the Heart

A person who suffered from a chronic cough or who had to constantly gasp for breath or breathe heavily was seen as being afflicted by a "heart-worm." It was believed that heart palpitations or a racing heart (tachycardia) were caused by "thickness of the blood," a heart-worm chewing on the heart, or a stone hanging on the heart. The leeches (physicians) of the olden days,* who also healed with incantations, visualized this kind of worm as a being with antler-like horns on its head. Heartburn was also thought to be caused by the "pissing" of a heart-worm. Moreover, this heart-worm could be a worm of hate or envy, or some sort of "aetheric" worm that wears a person down. The leeches of the times used various anthelmintic plants, such as allium species like bear leek or alpine leek (*Allium victorialis*), which were known to repel demonic spirits.

---

*The archaic term for a doctor, "leech," comes from Old English *læce*.

Smudging with special plants such as mugwort, juniper, or nightshades such as henbane for their healing smoke was also effective against these worms. Other plants used as "worm medicines" included valerian, blackberry, stinging nettle, gentian, fir needles, ground ivy, St. John's wort, carrot leaves, tansy, sorrel, plantain, wood fern, and wormwood. All of these plants continue to turn up in the old herbal manuscripts that were produced in later times. Enlightenment doctors scoffed at these cures as being superstitious, since it was obvious that these plants generally did not cure a case of roundworm or tapeworm. However, the worms that these plants were meant to repel were not physical creatures but rather "spirit worms" or "elf worms." If during a serious illness the heart-worm comes out of the mouth, they claimed, death is very near.

Nightmares (Demons of the Night)

When a night-demon called an *Alb* torments a sleeper and sits on their chest, the victim has trouble breathing and is overcome with feelings of dread.* These are conditions that, from a modern perspective, might be seen as having some connection to a heart or circulatory dysfunction. In earlier times, the belief was that elfish spirits of a malevolent kind cause frightful nightmares. Sometimes, a spirit of this sort rides the sleeping person like a horse so that he or she wakes up the next morning sweating, exhausted, and panting with a wildly pounding heart. The *Alb* robs its victims of their vitality, and in the worst case, they can even suffer a sudden stroke (*Apoplexia* = "paralysis") and die. Harmful elves like the *Alb* are spirit beings that can appear in many and shifting shapes, as a tomcat, a marten, a black dog, a fiery horse or bird, or in a human shape as a woman with bird's feet or toad's feet or a little man with bulging eyes and a fat head. Folk medicine had many cures for such beings. Pentacles carved into the bedposts were believed to protect the sleeper from bad spirits; scissors were strategically placed in the bedstraw or

*The German word *Alb* (also *Alp* or *Elb*) is related to the English "elf." Other dialectal names for a night-demon of this sort include *Drude* or *Trude*, *Druckerle* (assailant), the Alemannic *Toggeli* or *Doggi* (oppressor), the Frisian *Walriderske* (hedge-rider), the Bavarian *Schratt* (howler) or *Hockauf* (sit-upon), and the Franconian *Trempe* (trampler).

inserted into the keyhole (facing outward) of the door to keep the bad spirits at bay;* or a hatchet was placed near the bed with the sharp end upward, the person was covered with a wolf's pelt, and incantations were chanted like the following "elf blessing" from Bohemia:

Alb, Alb, du bist geboren wie ein Kalb,
Alle Wasser musst du waten,
Alle Bäume musst du blaten,
Alle Berge musst du steigen,
Alle Kirchen musst du meiden,
Und ob du das wirst tun,
Derweil will ich gut ruhn.

Alb, Alb, you were born like a calf,
All waters must you wade,
All trees must you leaf,
All mountains must you climb,
All churches must you shun,
And while you do these things,
I will rest well.

It was believed one could command bad spirits to do tasks that are impossible and then have one's peace. One saying in Baden, Germany, went: *"Doggeli, wenn du chunnst, so bätt!"* (*Doggeli,* if you can, pray!) Of course, an evil spirit cannot pray. It was not only possible to banish such a spirit in this way, but one might also appease it by giving it some offerings, such as food that had been censed with holy smoke, a small bowl of oil or milk, or "three white gifts" (salt, flour, and egg).

---

*One day an old man appeared at the house where I live. He told me that he had lived there as a child. He said there were nasty "imp spirits" in the house at that time, which would wake people at night, especially guests. The old grandmother knew what to do. She hung a pot of urine over the fire so that the whole house began to stink of urine. Then she put some scissors in the keyhole with the blades pointing toward the outside. After that, the imp spirits never returned.

Someone who had been attacked or ridden by a nightmare could be helped with certain herbs that protect against the cruel elves of the night, either by drinking a tea or wearing an amulet. One plant that can be used against nightmares and which is safe to drink as tea is yarrow (*Alchemilla vulgaris*). Others are dried and put into satchels for protection, such as holy rope (*Eupatorium cannabinum*); black nightshade (*Solanum nigrum*); woundwort (*Stachys alpinum*); bittersweet nightshade (*Solanum dulcamara*); mistletoe (*Viscum album*); the spores of stag's-horn clubmoss (*Lycopodium clavatum*), which are called *Alp*-flour; southern wormwood (*Artemisia abrotanum*), also called *Alp* rue; and fumitory (*Fumaria officinalis*) (Marzell 1943–1979, V:10).

Nervous Heart

Another descriptive term with deep roots in folk medicine is for the illness that was known as *Herzgespann* or *Herzgesperr* (anxious heart or heart palpitations; literally "heart-cramps" or "heart-lock") and which could befall humans and animals, especially horses. The term described pains and unease that started in the stomach and spread toward the heart. These unpleasant feelings were often accompanied by a tremulous and palpitating heart and tension that constrained the breathing and the elasticity of the diaphragm. The condition occurs when the "heart sac"—or the "heart ribbon" (the pericardium), the "little sac in which the heart hangs in the body"—is strained (Hovorka and Kronfeld 1909, 67). This "heart sac" can lay in a hampering way against the ribs. The *Allgemeines Oeconomisches Lexikon,* a home encyclopedia from 1731, states that *Herzgespann*

> [occurs] in people, but mostly small children, [and] consists in a swelling of the body under the short ribs, which causes difficult and anxious breathing, as comes about from cold air; severe gas in the stomach; and similar such things that hinder the *motom diaphagmatis* (movement of the diaphragm). (Grimm and Grimm 1877, X:1246)

For this disease, the healing plant motherwort (*Leonurus cardiaca*) was used. In German this plant is itself also called *Herzgespann*.

The heart could also break due to grief in love, disappointment, or shock, or it could shrink to the size of a bean (Bächtold-Stäubli 1987, III:1803). The breaking of a heart could even be heard: it cracked like a dry branch being broken. In a song written in the sixteenth century, we read: *"Krach, jungh Hertz, und brich nicht, / Die ich will, begert meiner nicht.* (Crack, young heart, but do not break, / The one I want, wants me not). The Grimm's fairy tale *The Frog King, or Iron Harry,* tells how the prince's loyal servant rides back with him and the new princess in a carriage. Three times they hear a loud crack, and the prince asks what the sound is. The servant tells them that he had three tight bands wrapped around his heart so that it would not break during the time the prince was enchanted and was a frog. As they rode back home to the castle and the first of the three bands broke, the following conversation ensued (which then repeats two more times):

> "Harry, the carriage
> Is falling apart."
> "No, sir, from my heart
> An iron band fell;
> For my heart grieved sore
> When you were a puddock
> And sat in a well." (Grimm and Grimm 2004, 274)

Heart-Stroke, Elf-Stroke

A heart attack, a sudden cardiac death (*Apoplexia cordis*), as well as a stroke (*Apoplexis cerebri*), were literally seen as the "stroke" of hostile otherworldly beings, especially elves. Traditionally, elves—or similar types of beings such as the *Alb*, the *Elbbütz,* or the Scandinavian *hulder* (the "covered" or "enshrouded" ones)—are not at all like the light, fairylike, friendly creatures with dragonfly wings we find described in romantic nineteenth-century literature and which are still gushed about today by New Age enthusiasts. Although these supernatural beings are occasionally benevolent to humans, they often lead them astray or put them under a heavy spell. Elves can be seductively beautiful, unpredictable, and have a luciferian intelligence. A normal human being is hardly able to withstand their magic. In his *Table Talk* (*Colloquia Mensalia*), Martin Luther relates that his mother suffered from the influence of a neighbor woman who practiced black magic; because of this contact, she suffered from an "anxious heart and malevolent elves" (Bächtold-Stäubli 1987, II:759). Some magicians, sorceresses, and shamans know how to communicate with such beings.

For Holger Kalweit, a German psychologist and researcher of shamanism, these are not fairy tales or primitive, prescientific fantasies. His research has convinced him that the occult beliefs of the pre-Christian Europeans have a thoroughly real basis. According to him, elves live in an invisible parallel world—a timeless, spaceless, nonmaterial, and magical "plasma-dimension." They appear to humans in dreams and visions. They play with mortals and find it entertaining to manipulate and enslave them, to befuddle them or drive them crazy, but also to occasionally send them inspiration for new works of art or mystical inspiration. They instigate adventure and bloody wars, send diseases and plagues, but also sometimes healing and healing knowledge (Kalweit 2006, 76). This is how the pagan forest peoples in northern Europe saw it as well, especially the Celtic and Germanic peoples. Elves often kill people with their magic arrows, which are called elf-shot (Old English *ylfa gescot,* Norwegian *alfskud,* Danish *elveskud*). They are often jealous of especially beautiful children or youths, gifted singers and musicians, and kidnap them into their ethereal realm—meaning they die young.* The breath of the elves (Norwegian *alvgust, elfblaest*) was also feared, which would bring sickness or death; it was feared as much as their "shots," which could bring on sudden death (Storl 2005a, 270; Storl 2018b, 179).

Fens and marshes were believed to be favorite places not only for

---

*When a particularly gifted and beautiful young person died, the hillbillies of Scotch-Irish background that I knew in the Appalachians would say that he or she was too good for this world, so the fairies took the young life.

witches but also for elves, such as the elf king and his bewitching daughters.* A Danish traditional ballad reworked into German by Johann Gottfried von Herder (1744–1803) and titled *Erlkönigs Tochter* (The Erl King's Daughter) tells us about Sir Olf, who was on his way to his bride when elves waylaid him. The charming Erl (Elf) King's daughter offers him her tender, white hand: "O, welcome, Sir Olf, to our jubilee! / Step into the circle and dance with me." Young lord Olf declines because the next day is his wedding day. He then declines the pile of gold the beautiful elf maiden promises, the two golden spurs, and the shirt "so white and fine, / was bleached yestreen in the new moonshine." Still, he answers: "I dare not tarry, I dare not delay, / To-morrow is fixed for my nuptial-day!" "Then, since thou wilt go, even go with a blight! / A true-lover's token I leave thee, Sir Knight." She "lightly struck her wand on his heart, / And he swooned and swooned from the deadly smart. / She lifted him up on his coal-black steed; / 'Now hie thee away with a fatal speed!'" He arrives "haggard and wan" and dares not get off his horse for fear he will drop dead. When his mother tells the bride what has happened, she cries out: "O, woe is me, Sir Olf is dead." The elf-shot, the heart-stroke, had hit him. (Translation from Mangan 1870, 215–18.)

HEALING INCANTATIONS AND HEART PLANTS

It was the task of the shamans, magicians, and leeches to ward off danger from the otherworld. They were visionaries; they could travel to the home of the elves and see the enshrouded elf being, or the "worm" or "evil spirit" of the disease, and they knew the powerful chants and magical, healing words. Sometimes they were able to bring back a stolen soul or ward off elf-shots.

Even after the conversion to the new religion of guilt and atone-

*The name *Elverkonge* (Elf King) from the original Danish ballad was mistakenly translated by Herder as "Erl King."

ment, there were still healers who continued to work in this way, only now they did so in the name of Christ. One of the important methods was to wipe off, or pull off, disease. There were women who had healing hands with which they could wipe off what had been conjured onto, or into, someone. There was also the method of pulling someone through a tree split explicitly for this purpose to "wipe the disease off." The tree then absorbed the disease. One could also hang diseases on the branches of trees, especially the elder tree. When doing this, it was important to recite a blessing, a healing charm. In Austria, there was a magical charm for a condition when the blood rushes to the head, accompanied by a fever, "when the blood surges from the heart into the head."* Whoever was suffering from this should say the following, while looking at a living tree branch on St. John's Day (June 24):

> *Ich steh' auf Holz und seh' auf Holz,*
> *Auf frische grüne Zweig'.*
> *Du Heiliger Geist, ich bitte dich,*
> *Hilf, dass das Sausen schweig.*

> I am standing on wood and looking at wood,
> On a fresh, green twig.
> O Holy Ghost, I pray to you,
> Please help let the buzzing be.

The aforemention ailment of "nervous heart" was also addressed with a charm to be released from it: *Scher dich los von der Rippe wie das Pferd von der Krippe* (Cut yourself loose from my rib, like a horse from its crib [hay-box]). Or: *Herzgespann, ich tu dich greifen, fünf finger tun dich kneifen* (Nervous heart, I will grab you, my five fingers will squeeze the life out of you).

Similarly, a charm could be used to force a heart-worm to leave the sick person. This usually concerned an invisible, "elvish" worm—as

---

*This might refer to tinnitus and headache caused by high blood pressure.

Paracelsus called it, a "worm without skin and bones, without a body and substance"—that was to be driven out. Here is an example of such a charm from ninth-century Bavaria, called *Gang uz Nesso* (Go out, worm!):

> *Gang ut nesso mit nigun nessiklinon,*
> *ut fana themo marge an that ben*
> *fan themo bene an that flesg*
> *ut fan them flesgke an thia hud,*
> *ut fan thera hud an thesa strala.*
> *Drohtin uuerthe so!*

> Go out, worm, with your nine little worms,
> Out from the marrow to the bone
> From the bone to the flesh
> Out from the flesh to the skin,
> Out from the skin into this arrow.
> Lord, make it so!

After the worm had been chanted into the arrow, it was shot off into never-never land. This is a genuine shamanic practice. Later worm charms threaten the worm with suffering such as Jesus Christ or his mother had to suffer, or the worm was required to accomplish an impossible task.

> *Herzwurm, ich gebiete dir bei Gottes Gericht,*
> *dass dich sollst legen und nimmer regen,*
> *bis die Mutter Gottes zweiten Sohn tut gebähren.*

> Heart-worm, I command you by God's Judgment,
> that you shall lie down and never move,
> until the Mother of God bears a second son.

Or the worm was banished, as in the following charm:

Unsere liebe Frau ging über Land,
Da begegnete ihr der Herzwurm.
"Ei, Herzwurm, wo willst du hin?"
"Ich will in das Nibhaus,
Will ihm sein Fleisch und Blut saugen aus."
"Ei, Herzwurm, das sollst du nicht tun,
Du sollst gehen in den grünen Wald,
Darin steht ein Brünnlein vor kalt,
Daraus sollst du essen und trinken,
Sollst nimmermehr des [Name] sein Fleisch und Blut
gedenken.
Amen." (Hovorka and Kronfeld 1909, I:455)

Our dear Lady was roaming the countryside,
and there she met the heart-worm.
"Hey, heart-worm, where are you off to?"
"I am headed to the neighbor's house,
I want to suck out his flesh and blood."
"Hey, heart-worm, you shouldn't do that,
You should go into the green wood,
There is a spring that is very cold,
You should eat and drink from it,
You should nevermore think of [Name], of his flesh
and blood.
Amen."

According to traditional northern European beliefs, the healing takes place through "word and wort." "Word" meant the magical charms and incantations that could penetrate into the deep, dark
recesses of the body and—by the strength of their virtue—force the
demons of disease, worms, or elvish beings to leave. "Wort" meant
the healing herb, root, or bark. In other words, the shamanic healing by chanting was accompanied by the practical healing with the
appropriate plants. Healing plants were sought that could destroy the

heart-worm's nest and kill it. There were various plants used for this purpose that differed from region to region. In western Bohemia, for example, the fresh juice of field scabious (*Knautia arvensis*) or of watercress was used. Generally, for heart pain and tremors, a poultice of oat flour, mallow, and henbane leaves was applied to the chest (Hovorka and Kronfeld 1909, I:68). Poultices of lemon balm were also applied. Common bugloss or alkanet (*Anchusa officinalis*) tea or common knotweed (*Polypodium vulgare*) macerated in wine was imbibed. Marjoram oil was rubbed on the nose. These are some of the many cures suggested for heart pain.

HEART DISEASES IN MONASTIC MEDICINE

By the later medieval period, when the Germanic-Celtic healing tradition had long since melded with the ancient teachings of monastic medicine, a person suffering from heart disease was described as one who could not eat *heartily,* laugh *heartily,* or love *heartily.* Someone who was always grumpy, sullen, or dejected was considered to have heart problems. Such a person was then given herbs and flowers that brighten and cheer the sense of well-being.

In the monastic literature of medical recipes, specific medicines for heart ailments are rare (Frohn 2001, 141). According to monastic medicine, what was dangerous to the heart were "rising vapors" in the body, which caused the pulse to become soft and slack due to overwhelming humidity. This could even increase to syncope, the sudden loss of power including passing out, cold sweats, and an extremely weak pulse. The monk/patient was then laid on his back, shaken, and his face was sprinkled with cold water; they tried to make him sneeze, twisted his fingers, and pulled some hair out as ways to bring him back around. Recurrent violent palpitations (*Palpitatio cordis*) were attributed to malignant vapors rising from the spleen into the heart. One then tried to eliminate these vapors from the spleen and to administer heart-strengthening medicines (Ingo Müller 1993, 277). Monastic medicine recommended the following herbal remedies for disturbances in the mixture of the bodily humors that affect the heart.* Only a few of these medicinal plants are native to northern and central Europe. They had to be cultivated in walled monastery gardens, protected from the cold and wind. Others are expensive spices imported from the Orient. From the modern scientific perspective of an active substance analysis, only a few of these plants—namely, motherwort, lily of the valley, and lemon balm—have a physical effect on the heart. They are listed here according to their medieval Latin names, which are given first.

CARDIAC REMEDIES IN MONASTERY GARDENS

Acetosa (*Rumex acetosa,* sorrel). The cooling and drying sorrel plant, which lessens the heat of bile and protects the heart against febrile illnesses and "rotten fever" (*febris putrida*), was often planted in the monastic *hortulus* (garden). Sorrel seeds, especially when collected by chaste virgins and carried as an amulet in a sachet, were said to protect the monks from nocturnal ejaculation. The arrow shape of the leaves was taken as a symbol of the martyrdom of Jesus. The leaf was also interpreted as heart shaped and thus, due to this signature, as a cardiac medicine (Gallwitz 1992, 211).

Basilicum (*Ocimum basilicum*). The warm, purifying basil plant has been used since ancient times as a tonic for anxiety, insomnia, cramps, and nervous discomfort; it was used to strengthen and cheer the heart and eliminate the malignancy of poisons.†

---

*These indications are based on the work of Ingo Wilhelm Müller and reflect the ideas of humoral galenic medicine. In traditional folk medicine, as well as in modern phytotherapy, these medicinal plants are used differently.

†The humoral medicine of the Middle Ages (with which Hildegard of Bingen was also familiar) prescribed remedies according to empirical-phenomenological criteria, or "qualities." Medicinal plants were thus "spicy," "sour," "greasy," "bitter," "salty," "sweet," "tart," "tasteless," and so on. In addition, they were characterized as warm or cold, moist or dry, differing in these qualities by four degrees of intensity. For example, bistort (*Bistorta officinalis*) was considered cold in the third degree and at the same time dry in the third degree. In contrast, garlic was considered to be particularly hot (fourth degree) and dry (fourth degree). Pumpkins were considered cold in the second degree and humid in the second degree. This hot-cold distinction has remained part of Latin American folk medicine to this day.

Bistorta (Bistorta officinalis). The cold to the third degree and dry root of the European native bistort is supposed to protect the heart against poison. It is also known as snakeweed.

Borago (Borago officinalis). The flowers and leaves of borage are believed to be cleansing. Since the plant balances melancholy and moderates acidic yellow gall, it also strengthens the heart and cheers the mind. Because borage lends the heart the courage of a lion, the herb was collected when the sun was in the sign of Leo.

Buglossum (Anchusa officinalis). Common bugloss has a similar uplifting effect as does closely related borage. The rough-leafed plant strengthens the memory and the heart and cleanses the "spirit," which, according to the worldview of the times, is an ethereal substance present especially in the left heart chamber, the arteries, and the brain chamber.

Calendula (Calendula officinalis). The marigold, which is native to the Mediterranean region and is considered warm and dry, opens and closes its golden-yellow-orange flower blossoms in a twelve-hour, day-and-night rhythm, and thus has a clear correlation to the sun. And, again, because the sun is the "planet" that governs the heart, marigold is considered a cardio-strengthening plant. With its yellow signature it also belongs to Jupiter, who governs the liver, protects against poison, and encourages sweating.

Cardiaca (Leonurus cardiaca). The warm, dry motherwort, also called lion's tail, gives the heart the strength and courage of a lion. In the *Gart der Gesundheit* (Garden of Health; Lat. *Hortus sanitatis*), an early herbal published by Peter Schöffer in Mainz in 1485, it was prescribed for stomach ailments, heart cramps, and tight-chestedness.

Carduus benedictus (Cnicus benedictus). The bitter-tasting, yellow-flowered blessed thistle is also classified as warm and dry and is said to strengthen the heart. Like the related milk thistle, this plant was generally considered good against "stitches (stabbing pains) in the heart."

Caryophyllus (*Syzygium aromaticum*). Clove, introduced from the Orient, also warm and dry in each case up to the third degree, was used to strengthen the brain, heart, stomach, and uterus.

Cerasus (*Prunus* spp.). Cherry, which was considered rather cold and dry in the humoral theory, strengthens the stomach, heart, and brain and cools fever. A symbol of eroticism, the cherry, in the sinless hand of Mary, becomes a sign of a sober, chaste heart.

Cinnamomum (*Cinnamomum verum*). Like clove and other expensive imported spices, cinnamon particularly pleases the heart when it is put into gingerbread dough. After it became known in Europe during the Age of Exploration, cinnamon nearly gained the status of a cure-all. It was said to improve the efficacy of spirits (alcohol), strengthen the heart and stomach, and expel poison.

Crocus (*Crocus sativus*). Expensive saffron, obtained from the stigma of the flowers of this member of the iris family, was believed to have practically the same medicinal properties as cinnamon. In Christian iconography, saffron yellow symbolized divine love and, because the heart is the seat of love, saffron was considered good for the heart.

Dictamnus (*Dictamnus albus*). The plant known as burning bush is full of essential oils; has a warming, drying, extracting (discharging, menstruation-promoting) effect; strengthens the heart; and protects against poison.

Lilium convallium (*Convallaria majalis*). The may bell or lily of the valley, which symbolizes the immaculate conception of Mary and is at the same time an attribute of the Christ Child, already delights the heart due to its fragrance. As late as the sixteenth century, Hieronymus Bock recommends a spoonful of distilled "may-bell flower water" in his *Herball or Generall Historie of Plantes* (1597) to comfort the heart; it is claimed to bring back "lost senses." A sneezing powder was also prepared from the plant, which helped one to sneeze out evil spirits hiding in the body.

Malum punicum (Punica granatum). The astringent pomegranate is believed to staunch bleeding and "fluxes" (catarrh, effusions, rheumatism, and secretions of any kind), reduce pungency, moderate bile, and thus also strengthen the heart and stomach.

Melissa (Melissa officinalis). Lemon balm has always been grown in monastery gardens and was a comforter for hysterical nuns. Hildegard of Bingen, who calls this mint *Binsuga* (bee-suckle), writes: "Whoever eats it will readily laugh because . . . the heart becomes joyful" (Marzell 2002, 205). It drives out black bile, neutralizes poisons, and strengthens the brain, nerves, uterus, and, of course, the heart.

Nymphaea (Nymphaea alba). The cool water lily, according to humoral theory, expels malignancy from the soul, cools fever, and strengthens the heart. In the monasteries, the water lily was used as an anaphrodisiac—that is, to quell the lust of the flesh and to expel lustful dreams that excite the heart.

Ribes (Ribes nigrum, R. rubrum). The effect of black and red currant leaves, whose medicinal use goes as far back as old Arabic culture, is described as cool and dry. The tea made from these leaves calms fluxes, reduces the heat of bile, and helps with diarrhea, fever, putrescence, and heart disease.

Rosa (Rosa gallica, R. centifolia, R. corymbifera). The red rose, an attribute of Mary and the symbol of love, was thoroughly connected with the heart during these times. Rose oil and rosewater from the petals were considered purifying, cooling, and strengthening for the heart, brain, spirit, stomach, liver, and spleen.

Rosmarinus (Salvia rosmarinus). The strongly fragrant and widespread rosemary herb, native to the Mediterranean countries, was considered not only anti-demonic but also rejuvenating, clarifying for the mind, and strengthening for the heart, senses, and brain. Rosemary wines and baths do, indeed, stimulate the circulation.

Veronica (Veronica officinalis, V. chamaedrys). Speedwell was believed to protect against contagion, to act as a sudorific, and to strengthen the heart. This plant under the protection of St. Veronica, who is said to have given Jesus the cloth to wipe his sweat while carrying the cross, "removes poison from the heart and guides it through sweat out of the body," according to Hieronymus Bock.

Viola purpurea (*Viola odorata*). For the monks, the violet, a symbol of humility and modesty, as well as for the sufferings of Christ, was considered cool, with the ability to expel ascended black bile (melancholy) from the heart and brain, purify the mind, and strengthen the heart.

We find other herbal heart remedies from this period in the writings of Hildegard of Bingen (1098–1179), who lived in a time when the theory of the four body humors of the Roman physician Galen was the prevailing dogma. The talented Benedictine nun did not consider the remedies (*remedia*), like we do today, to be vehicles for certain active ingredients.

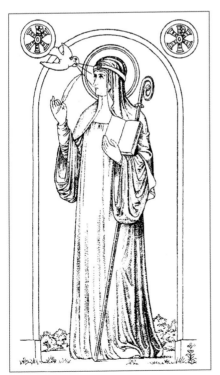

Hildegard of Bingen, the herbally enlightened nun

For her, the remedy (*remedium*), the medicinal plant, was always a medium or mediator of divine supernatural powers (Irmgard Müller 1993, 18). As a remedy for "heartache," she mentions plants that hardly affect the heart from a pharmacological point of view, including fragrant fennel (*Feniculum*), which is otherwise primarily known for digestion and respiratory organs; fenugreek (*Fenugraecum*), a phlegm drug; licorice root (*Liquiricuium*); the bark, leaves, and seeds of the sweet chestnut (*Castanea*); and black nightshade (*Solatrum nigrum*).

Some of the plants mentioned by Hildegard, such as the stomach remedy galangal (*Alpina officinarum*), yellow gentian (*Gentiana flavida*), and wormwood (*Artemisia absinthium*), are bitter-agent remedies. An old German proverb claims: "What is bitter for the mouth is healthy for the heart." Bitter substances have a positive effect on the circulatory system, even in the modern pharmacological sense. They not only stimulate the parasympathetic nervous system (vagus nerve) but also its antagonist, the sympathetic nervous system. Vagotonic people become more motivated, and sympathetic people can relax better. The heartbeat becomes a little stronger, the capillaries dilate, the vascular tone increases, and the coronary vessels become better supplied with oxygen (Bühring 2005, 80). Bitter drugs can thus enhance the mood and "warm the heart environment."

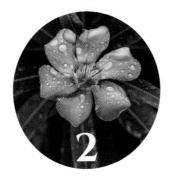

The Heart as the Abode of the Soul and an Organ of Perception

O how large is the liver, in which man's wrath resides,
and how small is his seat of love, this handful of a heart,
   by contrast!

Justinus Kerner (German medical doctor
and poet; 1786–1862), *Anatomische
Betrachtung* (Anatomical Observation)

Man must have earth under his feet, otherwise his heart
will wither away.

Gertrude von Le Fort

NOWADAYS WE CAN HARDLY IMAGINE what is meant by the word *soul*. For the most part, the concept of soul is replaced by psyche (from Greek *psukhē,* meaning "waft" or "breath," as the carrier of consciousness), which has somehow mainly become understood as a function of the brain. Early northern European peoples compared the soul to a lake (or to the sea) whose water can be in motion, churning, roiling, turbid, dark, or clear and calm, just like our own soul life, our feelings, drives, passions, emotions, and thoughts. The lake can also be placid and so smooth that the sun, the moon, and the distant stars are reflected in it. Indeed, the word *soul* is etymologically connected to the word *sea*. In a quiet soul, the spiritual archetypes and the invisible inhabitants of the inner side of the world can be reflected. The ancestors, deities, elves, nature spirits, and demons can show themselves in this inner (lake) mirror—which is found in the heart.

MOST DEFINITELY MORE THAN JUST A PUMP

According to Paracelsus, the heart perceives astral light. By this he meant that it intercepts the cosmic and orderly radiations of the stars—the celestial, or spiritual, impulses—and then passes them on into the blood. Thus, the heart is a perceptive organ. It is, therefore, as Aristotle put it, a seat of perception—in the literal sense of "hearing, grasping, understanding." What the heart perceives, the brain must then try to understand. Thus, the mind is associated with the head, the brain, but perception is associated with the heart. Already in antiquity, the heart was considered the seat of feelings and religious sentiments. For Empedocles, even the power of thought has its origin in the heart, and for Aristotle the heart was the "unmoved mover" (that which moves without being moved itself). According to church father Augustine, the Creator has written his law into the heart of man. The conscience, the inner voice, resides in the heart. For Pascal, the heart is the organ of inner feeling: "'Heart-knowledge' (*logique du cœur*)," he said, "gives immediate assurance in both philosophical and religious knowledge" (Schmidt and Schischkof 1978, 267). And the poet Friedrich Schiller states: "Your judgment can err, but not your heart."*

Hildegard of Bingen, whose worldview was a felicitous synthesis of the Christian-Mediterranean and old Germanic traditions, regarded the heart as the home of the soul. She compared the organ to the warming

---

*"*Dein Urteil kann sich irren, nicht dein Herz*" (*Die Piccolomini*, V:1).

hearth fire at the center of the house. "The soul lives in the heart as in a house; it sends its thoughts in and out, like through a door, and reflects on this and that as if it were looking through a window" (Hildegard of Bingen 1957, 167). According to her, thoughts rise like smoke through a chimney from the warm heart to the cool brain, and there they are transformed. Only after the fire of the heart joins the coolness of the brain can equanimity of thought result. Elsewhere, the enlightened nun says that the heart is the foundation of life and the location of the knowledge of good and evil.

According to an old German proverb, the heart hears more finely than the ears and sees more clearly than the eyes.* For the inspired poet Novalis (Friedrich von Hardenberg), the heart is the key to the world and life (Novalis 1980, 60). And, for Rudolf Steiner, the heart is a "sense organ for perceiving inwardly" (Steiner 1961, 38). The whole world is

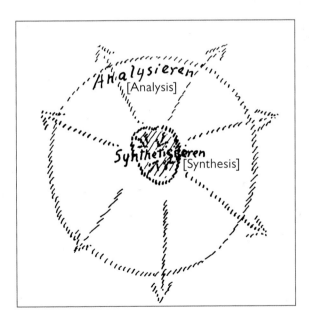

"The heart is the complete inverted image of the universe, contracted and synthesised." (Chalk sketch by Rudolf Steiner from Lecture VIII of *Geisteswissenschaft und Medizin* [*Spiritual Science and Medicine*, 1920])

Das Herz hört feiner als die Ohren; sieht schärfer als die Augen.

concentrated in this middle point; that which is scattered around externally as the universe is focused into a single point in the heart (Steiner 1961, 172). In other words, the whole universe is enclosed in the heart. Here, within the heart, in a pulsating exchange, the air we breathe in from the outside flows in and affects the blood that is circulating inside. Here, in a rhythmic balance, the macrocosm and the microcosm meet. According to Steiner, the constantly circulating bloodstream is briefly interrupted in the heart; it congests momentarily to take up, with the incoming breath, the etheric life forces and influences of the starry cosmos and then goes back into circulation. The heart is certainly not a pump; rather, the pulse of the cosmos is what causes it to move. In this way, the purely vegetative life of the body is "astralized" (from the Greek *astēr*, "star") and animated with star power so that consciousness can develop. In that it perceives this cosmic flow, the heart can be called a "perceptive organ" (Reinhard and Baumann 1992, 257).

The Heart as the Abode of the Soul

Different cultures entertain diverse views regarding where the soul—the dream self, the invisible doppelganger—is in the human body. Indeed, every part of the body can be considered the seat of the soul: spleen, liver, kidneys, or even the breath. Mostly and universally, however, it is the beating heart and the pulsing blood that is called the abode of the soul. The heart is called *inima* in the Romanian language, which goes back to the Latin *anima* (soul). In Welsh, the heart is called *calon;* like the Latin *caldus,* it means "warmth," because only that which is animated has warmth, has a warm heart. Elsewhere—for example, among the Lacandon people, who are descendants of the Mayan Indians from the rain forest in the Mexican state of Chiapas—the heart is considered the abode of the soul. The ethnologist Christian Rätsch, who lived with this tribe for three years, writes:

> The soul of man dwells in the heart. It is the nonmaterial duplicate, which leaves the body at night and acts in the usually invisible world in which almost everything is reversed, like in a mirror. The human

being perceives what the soul experiences as a dream. The soul can also leave the body in states of illness and visibly appear to other people. (Rätsch 2002, 446)

The Ojibwa, who populated the Upper Great Lakes region of North America, tell of a similar experience. For them, the soul has its seat in the heart, and, while a person is sleeping and dreaming, it can leave the body for a short time. If it does not return in due time, illness and ultimately death will follow. They also speak of black magicians, the Tcitaki medicine people, who have the power to hijack and capture the dream-soul of sleeping human beings, causing the victim to die (Hultkrantz 1992, 32).

For the Chinese, the body with its organs resembles a harmonious landscape where the seasons change. What matters is not the material organs but the dynamic relationships through which they are connected. The heart (*xin*), which controls the vessels and the blood, is empty, according to this view. It is a yin organ, receptive and incorporating. It is the prince of the organs. Like the emperor, it does not do anything. Thus, it can become the container of the spirit (*shen*). An old text (*Guan Junzi*) states:

> *Shen*—in heaven it is heat, on earth it is fire,
> in man it is spirit. (Heise 1996, 57)

A Chinese proverb says: "The radiance of the heart manifests on the face." *Shen* is the awareness that shines in our eyes when we are truly awake and fully conscious. If the heart supplies the body with sufficient energy (*qi*), then the person has a healthy complexion and clear eyes, emotional self-control, is confident, can concentrate and is well oriented, and thought and language are well ordered and full of meaningful content (Heise 1996, 10). The Chinese say: "The heart reveals itself in the tongue"—that is, in how one speaks.* If there is a lack of

---

*In German there is also an expression that literally translates as "to wear your heart on your tongue." "To wear your heart on your sleeve" expresses the same sentiment in English.

heart energy (*xinqi*), then a lack of concentration, forgetfulness, sleeplessness, and heart palpitations may follow. If an excess of fright, joy, fear, or another emotion inflames the mind, unrest will enter the heart. Restlessness and a disorderly agitation overpower the person; the face turns red, perspiration ensues, language becomes unclear, and there are uncontrolled or aggressive emotional outbursts. As a harmonizing agent for the heart, the Chinese use ginseng (*Panax ginseng;* Chinese *jen-shen*), meaning "human root" or "crystallized essence of the earth in human form" (Fulder 1985, 229). But there are also other remedies— such as jiaogulan (*Gynostemma pentaphyllum*), the so-called southern ginseng; or *xiancao,* the herb of immortality, which is now popular in alternative-health circles. Jiaogulan, a frost-hardy member of the pumpkin family, is practically a panacea but is said to be particularly good for the heart and circulation.

The Language of the Heart

We really do not know how our pagan ancestors conceived of the heart because there are so few written records that have been preserved. Much of the original culture has been erased or cleansed by zealous missionaries, priests, and their accomplices. Nevertheless, we can sense some things when we enter into the morphogenetic field (in the sense of Rupert Sheldrake) and listen with our hearts, as it were. Fairy tales, old folk songs, and proverbs contain traces and hints. But it is our use of language (especially with respect to idioms) that shows how the heart has always been considered the center of the soul's feelings and its place of residence. Following are some of the many "heart phrases" in English.

The heart can *take wings, stand still, sink, jump for joy, race, bleed for something or someone, be heavy,* or *be crushed.* One can *take heart, have a heart, unburden one's heart, rip into the heart of something, bare one's heart, pour one's heart out, sadden someone's heart, set one's heart on, lose one's heart to, follow one's heart's calling* or *follow one's heart, have heartfelt sympathy, not have the heart to do something* ("*my heart just wasn't in it*"), *do something halfheartedly, take someone into one's heart, lacerate the heart, take something to heart, heartily agree* (or *disagree*), *have someone near and dear to one's heart, have a soft spot in one's heart for someone, have one's heart in one's mouth, break someone's heart, be brokenhearted* or *heartbroken, love someone with all one's heart, have a heavy heart,* and *approach something wholeheartedly* or *halfheartedly.* One can *have a big heart, a warm heart, a soft heart, a cold heart,* even *an ice-cold heart, a wicked heart, a happy heart, an overflowing heart, give someone one's heart, touch someone's heart, have a heart for something or someone, entangle one's heart,* and *take heart.* An event or an occurrence can be *heartwarming* or *disheartening.* Something can be *heart-rending, the heart can "sink down to one's feet,"* one can *open one's heart to something.* Expressions such as *absence makes the heart grow fonder,* something coming *from the bottom of the heart, wearing one's heart on one's sleeve, with all one's heart, young at heart, tugging at the heartstrings, cross the heart and hope to die, have the heart in the right place, let your heart be your guide,* and so on—all of these idioms show just how deeply embedded the heart is in our world of feelings and how we express them.

In these sayings we can perceive that the heart has traditionally been seen as the midpoint of our feelings and the main place to express their depth. Similar examples can be found throughout the languages of Europe. Here are literal translations of some expressions from German: a mother carries a child *under her heart,* someone is *locked into someone else's heart* (loved very much), *to press someone to one's heart* (to hug), *to weigh something in one's heart* (to deliberate), *ensnarl one's heart* (lose one's heart hopelessly in hate, passion, or guilt), I say this with *my hand on my heart* (I swear it is true), *to carry a burden in one's heart, to place something in someone's heart* (ask him or her to take care of an issue), and *to do something with heart-blood* (passionately) (Röhrich 2001, 704–8).

HEART TRANSPLANTS AND CYBORG HEARTS

Some years ago, a heart-transplant procedure was shown on television. Viewers could see how the beating heart was operated out. At the same time, a donor heart—thoroughly chilled and temporarily immobilized with a potassium chloride injection—was on its way by special delivery. Would the helicopter arrive on time? The concern of the specialists was that too many heart cells could die during transit. The patient, a nine-year-old boy, was connected to an artificial heart machine and in a deep coma. For a very brief period, he was literally "heartless."

Finally, the cold heart arrived. The surgeons wasted no time trans-planting it. The donor heart began to beat. The operation was success-ful. An elderly doctor brought the redeeming message to the parents, who had been waiting, desperately hoping, and going through a grueling time in the waiting room: "The child is alive," said the angel of mercy in white with a thin-lipped, sympathetic smile. The best medical system of all time had, yet again, not been a letdown.

On December 2, 1982, at the University of Utah Hospital, a sixty-one-year-old dentist named Barney Clark underwent a seven-hour operation in which he received an artificial heart. The new organ was named Jarvik 7. Poor Barney survived 112 days without his original heart. The tubes in his chest, attached to an air compressor the size of a washing machine, caused constant inflammation. In addition, blood clots formed in the pumping mechanism, causing the patient to suf-fer numerous strokes. Since then, cardiac technology has obviously pro-gressed, not least of all with the help of NASA scientists. The artificial heart, which was implanted in Berlin in December 2006 into a forty-one-year-old patient, had an external power supply and control unit the size of a shoulder bag. Two replaceable batteries and a computer connec-tion were included.

Artificial hearts are essential for bridging the waiting period for a donor heart. Survival rates of up to eighteen months have been achieved with artificial hearts. As the supply of donor hearts is becoming increasingly scarce, these artificial hearts play an increas-ingly important role. The latest models are designed for a gestation period of up to seven years. In the United States alone, 2,192 donor hearts were transplanted in 2005, compared to 2,125 in 2006. The survival rate after one year is about 86 percent, up to five years at about 70 percent (WebMD 2020). In fact, heart transplants and artificial hearts are the conclusive proof that the heart cannot be the seat of the soul, the intelligence, or the emotions. It is merely a comparatively simple organ or a hollow muscle that, if defective, can be exchanged. This is reality. There is no room for unnecessary sentimentality or wistful projections. Or is there?

The Heart Remembers

Two physicians involved in heart transplants became aware of some strange phenomena. Dr. Paul Pearsall, a psychologist and specialist in neuroimmunology, and Dr. Gary Schwartz, professor of psychology and neurology at the University of Arizona, both noticed—independently of one another—that many of the patients with a new heart underwent a personality change. They took on many of the emotional qualities of their donors. It seems that there is a heart intelligence, as if the heart somehow stores memories. Here are some examples (Schwartz and Russek 1999; Sylvia 1997; Pearsall 1999):

- Pearsall reported that a woman who was relatively cold and dispassionate in bed before surgery became a nymphomaniac after her heart transplant. It turned out that the donor who had been killed in an accident had been a prostitute.
- A girl whose heart donor had been murdered kept dreaming of "her" murder in such clear detail that with her help the murderer could be found.
- A man with a donor heart tenderly called his wife by another name during sex; it turned out to be the name of the donor's wife.
- A former vegetarian developed a taste for beer, chili peppers, and chicken nuggets after the operation. As it turned out, these were the favorite foods of the heart donor. Another woman, a militant lesbian who had formerly enjoyed flipping hamburgers at McDonalds, suddenly loved men and became a vegetarian after receiving a new heart.
- Bill W., a businessman from Phoenix, was completely disinterested in sports before his heart surgery. When he recovered after the procedure, he became an avid extreme-sports athlete. The heart

donor had been a stuntman killed in an accident, whose leisure activities had been freestyle climbing and skydiving.

• An English truck driver named Jim, who did not care much for reading and writing and had barely graduated high school with bad grades, started writing long poems after he had a new donor heart. The heart donor had been a writer.

• A woman hated violence so much that she would even leave the room when her husband watched football. After her cardiac surgery, she not only watched football with enthusiasm but also began to curse like a sailor. Her heart donor had been a professional boxer.

• Following his heart surgery, a forty-seven-year-old man began to enjoy classical music and often spontaneously hummed classical melodies that he had never heard before. His heart donor was a seventeen-year-old violinist who been run over after a concert and died.

• Jerry was sixteen months old when he died, and his heart was given to Carter, whose age was almost identical to his own. When Carter was six years old, he met Jerry's parents. It was like he knew them. He ran up to Jerry's mother, hugged her, and rubbed his nose against hers just as Jerry had done. When she started to cry, he whispered to her: "It's okay, Mama." Then he hugged Jerry's father and called him "Daddy."

• A boy who got the heart of a drowned man developed a fear of water. Before the surgery, he was an enthusiastic swimmer.

These are just a few of the many examples of strange changes in behavior, as well as in the likes and dislikes, of those who have had a heart transplant. The physicians in charge try to ignore such mystical issues, which, of course, do not fit into their materialist worldview at all. But now researchers like Paul Pearsall, Gary Schwartz, and Linda Russek are studying these strange phenomena in more detail (Pearsall, Schwartz and Russek 2002, 191–206). In one out of seven transplant recipients they were able to observe and document such inexplicable transmissions. The organ recipients did not know their donors. Unlike the laws in Europe, the identity of the donor in the United States (different laws apply, depending on the state) may be disclosed. Therefore, it was easier to do this kind of research in the United States. Pearsall, Schwartz, and Russek concluded that the observed changes in behavior and preferences could not be coincidences; it just happens too often, and the details are too precise. Sometimes organ recipients discovered the donor's identity in an almost magical way, through unusual coincidences or lucid dreams.

But how can these mental pattern transfers of the deceased donors to the recipients be explained? The conventional answer is that the trauma of such a large-scale operation and the immunosuppressive drugs that the transplant recipients must take for their body not to reject the foreign organ cause profound changes in the personality. The fact that the organ recipient may develop certain patterns of behavior—new preferences, different eating and sexual habits, or the utterance of names that match people associated with the deceased donor—is seen as pure coincidence. Official doctrine claims that the function of memory obviously has its seat in the central nervous system, in the head, and nowhere else. Although a kind of memory regarding invading germs (antigens) can be attributed to the immune system, it contradicts scientific reason that transplanted organs should have a memory.

Pearsall and Schwartz cannot accept this dogma. Rather, they tend to theorize that it may be some sort of cellular memory, or that other body systems may be able to participate in such information and feedback loops (Pearsall, Schwartz, and Russek 2002, 191–206). While this does not yet say a lot, it is nevertheless significant, for it tentatively suggests that memory may be connected with more than just the brain alone. During the Enlightenment period in the seventeenth and eighteenth centuries, the brain was thought of as a kind of filing cabinet in which files with traces of memory were stored. Since then, progress has been made by comparing the central nervous system with the hard drive of a computer with bits of information stored on it. But is this really the case? Rupert Sheldrake, the internationally renowned biologist, mentions the frustration of neuroscientists who for decades have been unsuccessfully trying to locate memory in the brains of laboratory animals. Even if you remove large parts of the brain, the animals can sometimes still remember what they had been taught before the operation. Even in invertebrates such as polyps, which have no central nervous system but can still learn behavioral patterns, no precise seat of memory can be located. One of these researchers concludes that "memory seems to be both everywhere and nowhere in particular" (Sheldrake 1994, 116). This fact leads some scientists to assume that memory contents are stored in a nonlocal way. Sheldrake observes:

> But there may be a ridiculously simple reason for these recurrent failures to find memory traces in brains: They may not exist. A search inside your TV set for traces of the programs you watched last week would be doomed to failure for the same reason: The set tunes in to TV transmissions but does not store them. (Sheldrake 1994, 116)

Another question would be: "Who is sending the program, or from where is it sent?"

Confused Souls

All living beings with beating hearts and red blood have traditionally been considered to have a soul. They are "animated" in the sense of possessing an *anima* or *animus,* the Latin word for "soul." Hence ensouled living beings are called animals. Contemporary philosophers hardly dare touch on the subject of the soul, which is also referred to by some as the astral body. In psychology dictionaries one searches in vain for the word. If the soul is ever mentioned, it is in terms of a brain activity that is closely linked to hormonal, biochemical, and biophysical processes. But the soul cannot be reduced to brain functions. The whole body is animated. This means that we feel and sense—whether pleasure or pain, joy or suffering—with the whole body, from the scalp to the little toe. If the tip of the toe were not animated, it would not hurt to stub it or step on a tack; if the scalp were not animated, then a loving touch would not cause joy. Fingernails and hair, on the other hand, can be cut without it hurting, because they are not animated. A cow can eat grass and we can pick herbs without the grass screaming or the herbs trying to escape. This is because the grass lives like any other plant, but it is not animated. That does not mean that it has no soul; rather, it is surrounded by soul. The plant soul does not incarnate in its physical body but instead surrounds it and acts upon it from the outside (Storl 2013, 105). In humans and in animals, however, the soul is embodied, incarnating (from Latin *incarnare*, "becoming flesh") through procreation and birth.

We perceive and feel, we are moved, we have drives and emotions (from Latin *motio, movere, motum,* "move, excite, shake") because we have a soul. According to the traditional Western view, the soul is not some vague, undifferentiated, and misty entity, but it has certain centers in the body: the organs. Each body organ undergoes many experiences during a lifetime. Each organ experiences life in its own way. Most of the time, we are not aware of the experiences that our organs have because they are subconscious and subliminal. We do not know what experiences the liver stores or what impression sweets, intoxicating drinks, or certain emotions make on it. Also, the poisons—the physical as well as mental ones—that we swallow and which cause subliminal anger in us and possibly even cause the bile to overflow, belong to the biography of the liver.* If the liver is happy, then we are jovial.† The emotional residues of our social relationships are mirrored in our kidneys and urinary and reproductive organs; we literally absorb these feelings into our organs. Tensions and joys that connect us with spouses, neighbors, relatives, and enemies affect these organs and are stored psychosomatically; some of these things affect our kidneys. The lungs also have a biography. Our language reveals much about the amalgamation of the soul with the respiratory organ: sometimes we have to "catch our breath" or we are "left breathless," something can be "breathtaking," an atmosphere "suffocating," we "vent" our anger, we "let off steam." A German

---

*There is a German saying that (translated literally) asks: "What kind of louse crawled across your liver?" It is used in the same sense as the English expression "What's bugging you?"

†*Jovial,* meaning "cheerful, humorous," goes back to Latin *jovialis,* "belonging to Jove [Jupiter]." In antiquity, the god-king Jupiter was believed to rule over the liver.

doctor was convinced that it was above all the anxiety associated with air raids, flight from warzones, and other wartime horrors that had an effect on the lungs and then triggered the tuberculosis epidemics in the postwar years in Germany—because everything that affects the soul sinks down to the somatic level and manifests in the body. What gives true pleasure shows itself in the health and harmony of the body; that which hurts and saddens or terrifies the soul affects the liver, kidneys, spine, or some other organ or area of body tissue. This knowledge is the basis of psychosomatic medicine.

The same holds true for the heart, our central organ, the source of our life's rhythm: it also stores our intimate biography. Psychosomatic medicine shows that this organ is the focus of love, generosity, and courage. If you cannot open your heart, you constantly have the feeling of being constricted; in the long run this can turn into angina pectoris, a constricting feeling in the chest.* If you also lack nearby sources of love and human warmth, it can feel like you might as well drop dead. A subliminal rage, which causes the veins to swell, and the compulsive attempt to forcefully gain love and appreciation will raise the blood pressure. The soul works double time and loses its organic rhythm, its own ebb and flow of vital energy. The arteries become rigid, losing their elasticity, and the risk of a heart attack increases. Thus, the filtered-down negative psychic experiences influence the physical level (Tietze 1987, 73).

The heart remembers everything that moves it in life. For this reason, it makes sense that when one surgically removes the heart organ and transplants it in another person, the life experiences and heart memories of the former owner continue to resonate. It is no wonder that, as described above, many personality patterns can be transferred onto the recipient of the new organ. It seems practically inevitable. From the reports of those who have had transplants, we recognize that each body organ, not just the brain, is a carrier of consciousness. The function of the brain is simply to bring memories into everyday consciousness. In this sense, it is a mirror that reflects the deeper experiences—heart

---

*The word *angina* derives from Greek *ankhonē,* "strangling."

experiences, lung experiences, spleen experiences—much like the moon reflects the light of the sun.

This makes the utterances of organ-transplant patients, such as the following, understandable: "I began to feel that the spirit or personality of my donor lived on in me to some degree." "Sometimes I had the feeling that there was somebody else in me and with me, and that in some sort of indeterminable way, my ego-sense became a kind of 'we.'" "While I was not always aware of this extra presence, sometimes it felt like sharing my body with a second soul."

Dr. Pearsall reported that an eighteen-year-old heart donor who had died in a car accident had always liked writing poetry and songs. One year after the accident, his parents looked through the things he had left behind and found a song titled "Danny, My Heart Is Yours." In the song he talks about how he will die early, and his heart will be given to someone else. Indeed, the eighteen-year-old organ recipient's name was Danielle. She reports: "When they showed me pictures of their son, I knew him directly. I would have picked him out anywhere. He's in me. I know he is in me, and he is in love with me. He was always my lover, maybe in another time somewhere. How could he know years before he died that he would die and give his heart to me? How would he know my name is Danny?" (Pearsall, Schwartz, and Russek 2002, 194).

William Baldwin, a psychologist and reincarnation therapist, puts clients who have a transplanted organ into a light trance and lets them speak. Often, the dead organ donor expresses himself through the recipient. The psychologist writes: "The soul of the organ donor can follow the transplanted organ into the new body." He describes the case of Alex, from whom several donor organs were taken and who had the following words: "My kidneys went one way, my liver went another way, and my heart somewhere else. I followed my heart because that's where I live" (Baldwin 2003, 8–9).

These reports are shocking and raise questions that cannot be answered by our current mechanistic materialist worldview. There are many indications of old karmic relationships, of emotional ties that go beyond life. Also considered is the possibility of possession by the spirit of the deceased person to whom the organs once belonged. For shamans and seers, this is self-evident: even when a person dies, his or her spirit continues to exist independently of the brain in a nonphysical dimension. Burial rituals carried out by the community—washing and caring for the body, the wake, funeral feasts, ceremonial dances, and so on—help the deceased to shed the former body and move on to the path to the dead, to the ancestors, the gods, the stars, and out into the macrocosm. The dead are entreated to not remain—as ghosts—here on earth, but to move on, because the time has come to do so. One hands the corpse over to the earth, so that it—"ashes to ashes, dust to dust"—dissolves and releases the soul. Or it is cremated in fire, so that the soul may ascend in the smoke to the heavens. For Indian Hindus it is even forbidden to photograph the corpse so that the soul has nothing left in the material world to which it can cling.

But there are also cases in which the dead remain attached to the earthly realm. Occasionally, a soul is purposely prevented from leaving the community through occult practices, such as embalming or mummification, as was the case with Egyptian pharaohs or even today with the popes. The cult of holy relics works similarly. The soul is intentionally held back so that it can continue to be effective. South American Jivaros made shrunken heads (*tsantsas*) from the heads of their dead enemies with the purpose of capturing their spirit in the shrunken heads and using them as spiritual slaves.

It is different with those who were suddenly catapulted out of life by accidents. Often they do not realize that they are dead, and they wander restlessly in the nonphysical dimension (limbo). They frequently become ghosts, revenants, and energy vampires. Because they are bodiless, they try to slip into other bodies and take possession of them. If one's own heart beats and lives on in another body, then it is easy for the spirit to cohabitate that body. It is not difficult for a clairvoyant to recognize this form of possession. Such a case would be a challenge for a real shaman, who is able to visit the spirit world. They would have to convince the spirit of the deceased to let go of the past and the earth and move on into the light. Here, too, herbs help the dead soul on its journey. Hemp (*Cannabis indica*), for example, is a suitable psychedelic used by shamans to accompany the dead during their transition and help them find their way in the otherworld. The shamans of Central Asia and East Asia inhale the fumes of smoldering female hemp flowers for this purpose, a custom already described among the Scythians five hundred years before the Common Era. In West Africa, iboga bush (*Tabernanthe iboga*) helps contact the deceased. During cremations in India, the relatives of the deceased may eat bhang—fresh, crushed female hemp blossoms in yogurt—to help visually witness the passage of the deceased's spirit into a nonphysical dimension. In other cultures, there are other psychedelic herbs that serve this purpose.

In the case of restless or disoriented spirits of the dead, an incense made from dried mugwort (*Artemisia vulgaris*) and juniper sprigs (*Juniperus communis*) is helpful. These plants were already used by the ancient Germanic and Indo-European peoples during funeral rites. St. John's wort (*Hypericum perforatum*), blossoming in midsummer and bringer of much light, is also of great help as a fumigant. For the organ recipient, it is especially important that he or she sends thoughts of sincere gratitude and love to the deceased from whom the organ was received.

Artificial Hearts and Xenotransplants

Another question arises: What happens to humans when the new heart is no longer a genuine heart but instead a mechanical pump, an artificial heart, or TAH (total artificial heart) system whose electrical power source is a plug behind the left ear (rather than a longer cord piercing the abdominal wall, which is prone to infection). What are the psychological consequences? A subfield of anthropology called cyborg anthropology concerns itself with the meaning of artificial body parts—artificial hearts, prostheses, pacemakers, implants, and other inner-body technology—in living human beings.*

Cyborg refers to a cybernetic organism, a hybrid of a living organism and a machine. Technocratic optimists believe that the advances in cyborg technology will continue to improve the body's attributes and help overcome human limitations.

The same question arises in what are called xenografts—that is, transplantations of hearts from other mammal species into humans. Because human donor hearts are often in short supply, the hearts of our closest relatives, the chimpanzees and baboons, have been considered. In 1964 the first attempt was made at the University of Mississippi when the heart of the chimpanzee Bino was transplanted into the sixty-eight-year-old patient Boyd Rush. Unfortunately, the pumping power of the monkey heart was too weak and the patient's defensive reaction too strong, causing him to die after ninety minutes. Four years later, in London, a pig's heart was transplanted into a human body. The animal heart continued to beat for only two minutes. In 1984 a surgeon in California transplanted a baboon's heart into a fourteen-month-old infant named Fae. Although the surgeon had a lot of experience with transplanting hearts—he had also transplanted lamb hearts into children—baby Fae died after twenty days.

Nowadays, a lot of hope is riding on pigs' hearts. They are like the human heart in size and pumping capacity, and there is no risk of transmitting a human-compatible monkey virus. Chimpanzees are now a protected species, but there are plenty of pigs available. Except for Muslims and Jews, there are no religious ethical concerns with pigs. According to the FAO (Statistic 2002), there are almost one billion pigs worldwide, with 90 million slaughtered per year alone in the United States. The biggest problem with animal-heart transplantation is the immunological defense reaction of the recipient. Genetic engineers plan to mitigate this by breeding pigs with human genes. Other organs, heart valves, and skin can then be taken from genetically modified, cloned pigs.

If organs are bearers of the soul and psychic impressions, then the question arises as to what influence this could have on the personality of the person with a pig's heart. "Would he start grunting at lunchtime and act piggish?" an English friend asked with a wink when we discussed the subject. With typical British understatement, he then remarked that if this did really happen, no one would take much notice of it in today's world, anyway.

Asuras

Not everyone agrees with transplantation medicine. Jehovah's Witnesses reject the idea of cardiac and other organ transplants, claiming that if a person takes live organs from other people to continue a human life, it amounts to nothing less than cannibalism and is, as such, a grave sin. Some spiritually oriented people reject organ transplants because they believe that the ghosts of the deceased owners are still here on earth as so-called earthbound spirits and will not be able to go to heaven. Not only does this hinder them from moving on spiritually, but they may also remain in the organ recipient, causing the latter to become possessed.

A few years ago a friend of mine, a farmer-philosopher named Arthur Hermes, commented on organ transplantation. He said that Rudolf Steiner had predicted that, at the end of the twentieth century, spiritual beings, which he called Asuras, would rise from the very foundations of creation and attack humanity.* They would not, like the Ahrimanic forces, lead to one-sided, coldhearted intellectualism, nor would they, like Luciferian forces, distract humans into dreamy, aesthetic illusions, but they would literally—through the actions of doctors who are possessed by them—tear away and devour, bit by bit, the soul parts of humans (and animals).† These would then be irrevocably lost. What then remains are mentally castrated people who are trapped in their lower, instinctive nature, people who only believe in physical matter. Materialistic black magicians who receive inspiration and power from the Asuras then have no inhibitions about cutting (harvesting) living organs out of bodies,

---

*The term *Asura* (Sanskrit *asura,* "demon, evil spirit"; as an adjective, "evil, devilish"), which Steiner borrowed from Theosophical vocabulary, designates a spirit of darkness. In the beginning the Asuras were equal to the gods, but over the course of time they decided to pursue their own selfish advantage instead of the truth.

†The terms *Luciferian* and *Ahrimanic* derive from Rudolf Steiner's philosophy, which is called Anthroposophy. They describe two types of seduction that draw people from their center, where, according to Steiner, Christ is found. Lucifer (light-bearer) is the fallen angel of light, the seducer who lures human beings into beautiful, unrealistic dreams and illusory worlds. Ahriman, named after the ancient Persian antagonist of the good god Ahura Mazda, rules over lifeless matter and the cold intellect; this principle seduces humans out of their naturally warm and human dimension.

aborting embryos, and mutilating the body as a soul carrier. These misguided scientists believe they are doing good things; they have no idea that they are remotely controlled by the Asuras and that it is something other than their own personal ideas that motivates them.

When Arthur Hermes told me these things, they seemed like wild sci-fi fantasies or weird paranoia. But who knows? Already in 1923, Rudolf Steiner gave a lecture for workers at the Goetheaum (Dornach, Switzerland) in which he said that cows would go insane if processed slaughter wastes were mixed into their feed. More than half a century later, scientists recommended that additional protein (from cadavers) in the fodder would increase milk yield and meat production—the result was the outbreak of Mad Cow Disease (BSE). In his lectures, the anthroposophist also pointed out that toward the end of the twentieth century, there would be a decline in human fertility in Europe. Did Steiner—a man known to be clairvoyant—perhaps also perceive something in other dimensions when he spoke of organ-eating Asuras?

DIABOLOS

We live in diabolical times. The word *diabolical* truly fits; it comes from the Greek *diabállein* (to set at variance, to set against). We really do live in times when what used to be ordered is jumbled, contentious, confused, and chaotic. It is happening at all levels: social and ethnic structures become ever more confounded, gender issues are chaotic, biological systems are becoming ever more jumbled, and species boundaries are bypassed through genetic engineering. For the aim of profit and with no holds barred, genetic engineering now splices genes from disparate lines of inheritance that developed over millions of years: firefly, flounder, and snowdrop genes in potatoes; laurel tree genes in rapeseed; artichoke genes in sugar beets; bacterial genes in corn; human genes in pigs; and much more. Even the ecological systems that have evolved naturally over long periods of time are being churned up, made chaotic, and their organisms are under unprecedented and extreme selection pressure. Exotic plant and animal species are conquering new territory and oppressing indigenous species. In Europe, for example, American raccoons are now robbing bird nests, bullfrogs are eating the spawn of indigenous amphibians, and North American muskrats and gray squirrels are spreading, as are the Chinese mitten crab and the raccoon dog from East Asia. Spanish slugs, American corn borers, and San Jose scale insects make their way through the crops. In the United Kingdom, the New Zealand flatworm is replacing native earthworms, thereby destroying valuable humus soil. Voracious Chinese ladybugs, introduced to protect plants from aphids, eat seven times as much as the native ladybug, which, because nothing is left to eat, starves. If they cannot find enough aphids, the Chinese beetles descend upon the grapes. In Europe, robust plant species from distant regions—invasive plants such as giant hogweed, Japanese knotweed, Canadian goldenrod, or Himalayan balsam from Kashmir—stifle indigenous flora. Conversely, Eurasian flora and fauna in Australia, South Africa, and America cause equally immense damage.

The social world is likewise in complete chaos: cultural patterns that have emerged over thousands of years in harmony with the natural environment are being disrupted. The traditional human cultures of the Asian steppes, the primeval forests and savannas of Africa, and the arid environment of the Middle East now meet up with—for better or for worse—the multicultural, global milieu of big cities. Can cultures be transplanted just like organs are? The traditional family, as a building block of traditional social organization, is increasingly being replaced by single households, patchwork families, same-sex relationships, and other alternatives. Even the language, the cultural bond of civilizations, which also links tribal societies to their natural environment and their history, is becoming globalized or "McDonaldized." Since the Eskimo in Alaska no longer speak Inuit but instead the language of a distant island in the North Sea, it is ever harder for them to survive by their traditional hunting. The indigenous words are missing to describe the various states of ice and snow, the behavior of marine mammals, and other conditions necessary for survival in their world of ice. The language of the colonial rulers has not grown organically in this specific environment and is not adapted to the landscape, the climate, and the way of life, as is the language of the natives. Languages are part of the ecology. With every language that goes extinct, the ancient, millennia-old wisdom of the ancestors is lost. Deeper connections can no longer be readily recognized and communicated (Nettle and Romaine 2000, 69).

The transplanting of organs and the international organ trade are also part of the diabolical zeitgeist, which, like a mental cyclone, shakes everything up. It seems as if the cards have been reshuffled, the field plowed to receive a new crop. It is the dance of angry Kali, the Shiva Tandav dance, the dance of destruction, the ever-faster dance of dissolution that precedes re-creation (Storl 2004a, 140–41).*

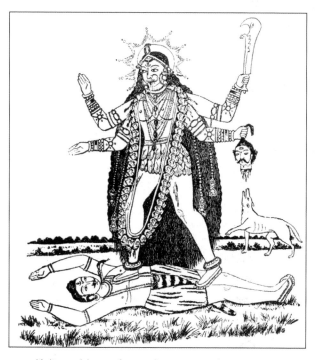

Kali, goddess of transformation, destruction,
and new beginnings

---

*Tāṇḍavam (also known as Tāṇḍava natyam) is a divine dance performed by the Hindu god Shiva. Shiva's Tandava is described as a vigorous dance that is the source of the cycle of creation, preservation, and dissolution.

THE MICROCOSMIC SUN

In the science of antiquity it was not the brain that was seen as the seat of the soul but rather the whole body with all its organs. This idea flourished again in the Renaissance with the teaching of the planetary gods. The universe was perceived as a weaving of invisible forces that pulse through the entire cosmos—the landscape, people, animals, plants, stones, metals, and the starry sky. The primal impulses came from the fixed stars, the twelve regions of the zodiac. Changed, interwoven, and mixed, these impulses were then further transformed by the seven (visible to us on earth with the naked eye) "moving stars," the planets. These celestial bodies were not seen as lifeless, rotating spheres of

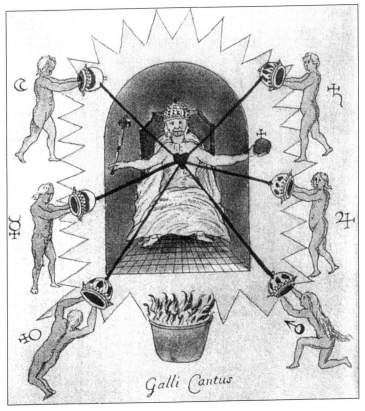

All organs and planets orbit the heart-sun.
(*La Sagesse des Anciens*, eighteenth century)

dust and matter but as deities. Above the sun are the so-called superior planets: Saturn on the edge of the fixed stars, then, respectively closer to the sun, Jupiter and Mars. Nearer to the earth are the inferior planets: Venus, Mercury, and the moon. Between the superior and inferior planets, the living heart of all greater nature, the sun, moves along the ecliptic, shining for all that exists. Each planet corresponds to an organ of the macrocosmic soul.

The human being, the small microcosmic world, mirrors the macrocosm. In humans, the heart is the sun. The major organs rotate their energies as inner planets around the sun. Here, too, everything is interrelated. The organs, the inner planets, pulse their energies throughout the whole body. In this way, the heart radiates its living light into the microcosm; it is the same light that shines back out through the eyes. Seen in this way, the eyes are the gateway to the soul, to the heart. Paracelsus writes (*Volumen Paramirum*, 1585):

> The heart is the sun, and as the sun shines on the earth and affects it, likewise the heart affects the body. And if this effect does not come from the sun directly, then it is from the body, for the body must have enough sun in its heart. Likewise, the moon can be compared to the brain, and the brain to the moon. (quoted in Rippe and Madejski 2006, 100)

The brain belongs to the moody, changeable moon; it is a sensitive silver mirror that reflects. The clever, devious quicksilver-like Mercury, which circulates the lymph and controls the mind, has its organ in the lungs. Lustful Venus has its seat in the kidneys. Mars, which gives courage but also anger, is connected to the gallbladder. Jupiter, the god of the fullness of life as well as of gluttony, is associated with the liver and gives dignity and maturity. Old Saturn, the slowest planet whose organ is the spleen, can embitter our soul, make it melancholy, or fill it with crystalline wisdom.*

*For more on these planetary correspondences, see Wolf D. Storl, *Culture and Horticulture* (2013) and *The Herbal Lore of Wise Women and Wortcunners* (2012).

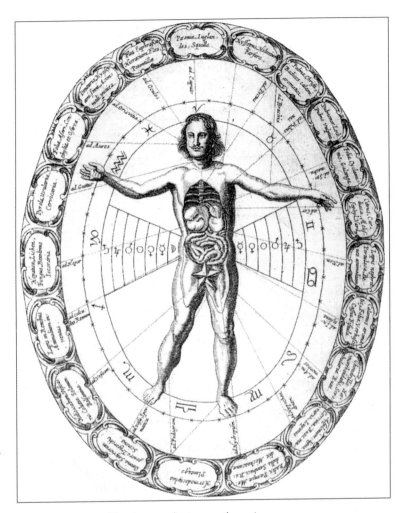

The human being as the microcosm
(Athanasius Kircher, *Mundus subterreaneus*, Amsterdam, 1682)

Other cultures also knew of such comprehensive, holistic systems in which the organs were described as bearers of psychic qualities. Traditional Chinese medicine (TCM), for example, speaks of the Seven Emotions (*Qi Qing*) (Ots 1990, 45; Heise 1996, 56). According to TCM, rage and aggravation accumulate in the liver. The kidney is prone to anxiety and fear. Grief, worry, or nervousness gather in the lungs. Anxious brooding has its seat in the spleen. And the heart, which can sense whether it is targeted with loving or hateful intentions, is prone to joy and fright.

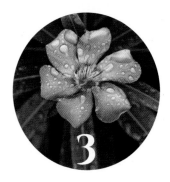

THE HEART AS THE SOURCE OF LOVE AND VITALITY

My heart is like the sea,
Has storms and ebb and tide,
And some beautiful pearls
Resting in its depth.

HEINRICH HEINE, *BOOK OF SONGS*,
"THE HOMECOMING"

The video screens are getting bigger, and the
hearts are getting smaller.

AMMA (SRI MATA AMRITANANDAMAYI)

THE HEART IS THE SPRING and sacristy of love. Our true self, the divine spirit, lives and thrives in the heart. Everything we love is directly connected to this center. The image of the one dearest to the heart, the companion perhaps through many lifetimes, remains well preserved in this innermost chamber, like a jewel. And then, when the eternal lovers meet on earth for the first time in this life, their hearts recognize each other. The heart is wiser than the mind. Two soul mates have now found each other. They have the key to unlock each other's heart. They give each other their hearts, or as it was said in the Middle Ages, they "exchange hearts." We know from ancient legends and fairy tales that this idea was a reality for the northern forest peoples who spoke Germanic languages, especially those of England and northern Europe.

THE HEART AND ETERNAL LOVE

Even the ancient peoples knew love affairs and unfaithfulness; married couples were divorced; bastards were begotten; passions were inflamed—the sagas are full of this. Such stories have nothing to do with the true heart's companion but instead with personalities—in the sense of Latin *persona* (mask of an actor). Personalities can marry, have sex with each other, accumulate possessions, manage their affairs, produce children (heirs), and even be happy throughout the marriage. How often, however, is the German saying appropriate: "The Savior had to suffer distress, disgrace, and shame, but he was spared one thing, and that was the life of a married man."* Personalities get caught up in social roles. By contrast, it is what lies at our core, the Self that dwells in the heart, that celebrates the sacred marriage (the *hieros gamos*). True marriages are made in heaven, not in the business of the everyday world. In German, the word for "marriage," *Ehe*, is distantly related to the word for "eternal" (*ewig*).† *Eternal* originally did not mean an infinite length of time but instead that which was beyond time—in heaven, in the divine, in immortality—located behind the veil of flowing time. These are certainly unrealistic dreams for the postmodern human, who stumbles from one relationship to another, lives as a frustrated single, falls in love again, only to be disappointed again, until s/he maybe finally finds a partner for life, or a life stage companion; or even for those to whom marriage is a kind of torture and a prison. But this precisely reflects a society that has lost access to the strength of the heart. A society in which the heart is understood only as a

---

*Der Heiland musste erleiden Not, Schmach und Schand', / Doch eins blieb ihm erspart, das war der Ehestand.
†The German word *ewig* is etymologically related to the Greek *aiōn* (lifetime, eternity) and the Sanskrit word *áyus* (Life force; according to Vedic interpretation life is not an epiphenomenon but instead a component of eternal being).

bio-cybernetic pumping organ; it is no longer a sacred space, the threshold to the divine and eternal, that it once was.

And yet, there is hardly a love song, or some new hit, that is not singing about the heart, *el corazón, le cœur.* (This brings to mind what a Pueblo Indian allegedly once said: "One sings about what one does not have but would like to have. White people sing about hearts and love, and we Hopi sing about rain for the fields.")

The Book of Eternity

It is a custom for lovers to immortalize their love by carving their initials in the smooth, lead-gray bark of old beech trees. A heart pierced by an arrow, with names or initials inside, is carved into the bark of the old tree. In this way, they write into the book of eternity that they have become soul mates. The beech belongs to the old, gray-bearded planet-god Saturn, the guardian at the blue, heavenly gate. He is imagined as carrying a thick book in which he notes everything that is to endure into eternity. In the night sky, Saturn appears as the last planet still visible to the naked eye. All the other planets orbit below Saturn's orbit, and beyond Saturn are the fixed stars, the home of the immortal archetypes. In short, below Saturn is the constant weaving and waking of the transient world, and beyond Saturn is eternity. We see that Saturn is the gateway to the divine archetypes. And because the beech participates in "Saturn essence," the tree is also a gateway to the divine realm.

Long before the medieval planetary doctrine came along, it was known that the gods can announce themselves in beech trees. The Celtic and Germanic seers and sages heard the whisperings of the Great Spirit in the rustling beech forest. And they carved what the gods whispered to them as runes into the gray bark of the beech trunks or onto cut branches, onto beech staves (German *Buchstäbe,* from which comes our word "book"*) They brought the carved runes to life by coloring them with fresh red blood or ocher. Then they threw the sticks onto a

---

*In German, the etymological connection between the two terms is fairly transparent: *Buch,* "book," and *Buche,* "beech."

white linen cloth, picked up some of them, and tried to infer divine will (Scheffer and Storl 2007, 162). The heart pierced by an arrow can be interpreted as one of the last remnants of such magical rune practices.

Cupid's Arrows

The arrow that comes out of nowhere, lands in the middle of the heart, and ignites it in love is an ancient motif in Indo-European cultures, and one that carries on to the present day. In a German folk song, "Im Wald, im grünen Walde, da steht a Forester's House" (In the Woods, in the Green Woods, There Stands a Forester's House), the lyrics speak of the "shot to the heart":

> Der Förster und die Tochter, die schossen beide gut.
> Der Förster traf das Hirschelein, die Tochter traf das
>   Bürschelein,
> tief in das junge Herz hinein,
> tief in das junge Herz hinein.

> The forester and the daughter, they both shot well.
> The forester hit the roe deer, the daughter hit the lad,
> deep into his young heart,
> deep into his young heart.

The archer is Cupid (or Eros), the god of love. It was Eros among the Greeks—to whose name we owe such words as *erotic* and *eroticism*. The young, winged shooter was born out of an amorous adventure between beautiful Aphrodite and the stormy warrior god, Ares.* The ancient Greeks regarded Eros as the embodiment of the sexual instinct itself; in Orphism, he was seen as the driving force of creation, which created the cosmos out of chaos. Much later, however, in the period of the Baroque

---

*Aphrodite, the mistress of sensual desire, was born at the dawn of creation, when Chronos created time and space by splitting the unity of heaven and earth, thereby castrating his heavenly father, Uranus. The divine god's member fell foaming into the sea, and Aphrodite emerged out of the foam.

and Rococo, the mighty god turned into the little naked, chubby cupids, or *putti,* who spurred frivolous society to erotic flirtations by shooting them with their arrows. The Roman equivalent of Eros was Amor (Latin for "love"), the son of Venus, who was also called Cupido (Latin *cupiditas,* "desire, suffering"). He also appeared as a winged youth with bow and arrow. The legend that surrounds him tells of a king who had three daughters. All three were lovely, but Psyche (soul) was the most beautiful. She was so beautiful that even Venus became jealous of her. The goddess, who wanted vengeance, sent her son Amor to confuse Psyche. He was supposed to use his sharp arrows and kindle in her love for an ugly old man. But when Amor saw beautiful Psyche, he fell in love with the lovely girl himself. Once, when she fell asleep, he abducted her with the help of Apollo and took her to a secluded, sacred mountain. When she woke up, she saw a beautiful golden castle before her eyes. As she stepped through the gate, she saw a table set with the most delicious food. Everything was decorated with flowers, and she heard beautiful singing, but she saw no one. When she got tired, she went into the bedroom and fell asleep. Then invisible Cupid came to her and gave her ten-

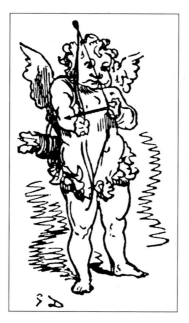

Amor
(Gustave Doré)

der love. This went on night after night. Every evening the invisible lover came to her. Psyche would have liked to see the person who made her so happy and intoxicated her senses. However, he had urgently warned her that if she looked at him with her own eyes, he would have to disappear and would never return. Psyche was very happy in the castle, although there were times when she felt lonely. She missed her sisters and invited them to visit her. They came but were envious of the splendor, and when they heard about her nocturnal lover, they thought it must be a monster. Why else would he hide? They advised her to get to the bottom of the matter. So, one night after he fell asleep, she secretly lit a lamp to look at him. Contrary to her anxious expectation of seeing a dragon or some other monster, she saw a beautiful young man. A drop of hot oil from the lamp fell on his shoulder, waking him. Then he became very sad and said that now he would not be able to come back. All her bitter tears were in vain. She searched for him for many years but could not find him. Cupid, too, desperately searched for Psyche. At last, they found their way to the mountain of the gods, where Jupiter, the king of the gods, appeased the jealous mother, Venus, and reunited the two lovers. In heaven, they had a lovely daughter named Epithymia, "sensual pleasure" (Grabner-Haider and Marx 2005, 112).

What does the myth mean? Many things, such as that the soul and sensual love belong together, but also that the bright light of the curious mind—sexologists beware!—dispels the wonder and the magic of erotic love and leaves the soul in solitude and sadness.

Cupid's arrows clashed with Christianity. In church imagery, if an arrow pierces a heart, it means a martyr's death. Since the time of the plague, the Blessed Virgin Mary has been depicted as the Mater Dolorosa (Mother of Sorrows), with a heart pierced by seven swords. Darts of ecstatic love for God, however, were not unknown in Christianity—a pierced, flaming heart is an attribute of the church father Augustine (354–430). Saint Theresa of Ávila (1515–1582), the founder of the order of Discalced Carmelites, had a vision of an angel piercing her heart with a burning arrow of divine love. In 1562, she celebrated a mystical engagement with Jesus. It is said that when she was struck by too much love-fire, she grabbed her tambourine and began to dance, and her sisters accompanied the rhythm with castanets and clapping hands. Theresa is, together with St. John of the Cross (1542–1591), a founder of the "Jesus Prayer," which in German is referred to as the *Herzensgebet,* "Heart's Prayer."

Luitgard, a Flemish girl from the twelfth or thirteenth century, had been put in the cloister at the age of twelve, where she saw a young knight at the age of fifteen and was struck by the arrow of the god of love. After this meeting, she did such hard penance that a vision revealed to her the divine bridegroom, Jesus. She fled, as it is recorded in her biography, into Christ's wound on his side and rested there like a child in a cradle. Through meditation on the Sacred Heart, sensual passion (*sexus*) and the interplay of expectation and surrender (*eros*) finally become true love (*agape*) (Beyer 1996, 147).

The Love Darts of Kama

In India, too, the beautiful young god with his quiver full of arrows is well known. There he is called Kama or Kamadeva (Sanksrit *kama,* "desire, longing"). The name is known to us in the West through the *Kama Sutra,* the ancient Indian textbook on the art of sensual love. It is said that Kama was the firstborn son to have sprung from the heart of the creator god Brahma. Others say he is the son of Lakshmi, the goddess of fortune, who, incidentally, rose out of the foaming sea, much like Aphrodite. Others call him Aja, "the one born of no one" or "the self-arising one." In the *Rig Veda* (X, 129, 4), the oldest written work of Indo-European origin, he embodies the first impulse of the Absolute:

> Thereafter rose Desire [Kama] in the beginning,
>   Desire, the primal
> seed and germ of Spirit.
> Sages who searched with their heart's thought
>   discovered the
> existent's kinship in the non-existent. (Griffith
>   1889–1892, II:575)

Kama bestows pleasure and joy and is a prerequisite for the emergence of all living beings, for generating new generations, no matter if they are humans, animals, plants, or gods. Shiva, the ascetic and god of gods, did not like this. He did not want to immerse himself in the maelstrom of passion, to be entangled in the wheel of illusion, the endless cycles of pleasure and suffering, birth and death. As a yogi, covered with ash, lost in deep meditation, he sat alone on the icy summit of Kailash, the world mountain. In silent contemplation, he meditated on the undivided foundation of being. He embodied pure consciousness and bliss; the fire had burned out in him, and there was nothing left but ashes. Because the great god was indifferent to the restless doings of the world, everything was chaotic on earth. Unhampered, demonic beings pursued their greed and lust for power. No one was there to protect the people, animals, gods and plants from abuse, exploitation, and suffering. The beleaguered creatures prayed to Brahma that they would be redeemed from the suffering and that their joy of life would return. Wise Brahma

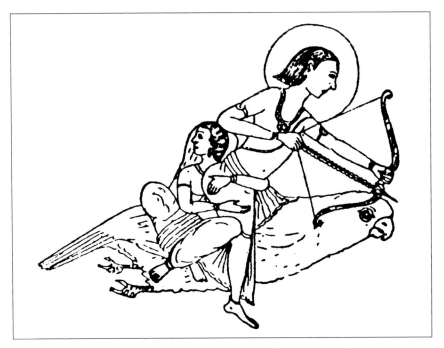

The god of love Kamadeva (Nepalese depiction)

told them that only a son from the god of gods (Mahadev, Shiva) could save the world. This son, divined Brahma, would one day be born of Shiva with beautiful young Parvati. But how could that come to be? Shiva was inaccessible; he had extinguished every emotion within himself through extreme asceticism.

Parvati, the lovely daughter of the mountains, conferred with Brahma and the other gods. They decided to send Kama. He should shoot a love arrow directly into the heart of the ash-covered ascetic. Kama seized his bow made of sugar cane, with its string that hummed like bees swarming around honey, packed the flower arrows into his quiver, and settled on the colorfully feathered parrot, which was his mount. This was how he flew to the rugged mountain. Gentle, warm air followed him, and the land he flew over began to turn green; birds sang spring songs, and colorful flowers sprouted out of the earth. A band of celestial dancers, *apsarasa*, accompanied him, and the cuckoo bird (in all of Eurasia known as the messenger of spring) also announced his arrival. Parvati and the gods also joined this happy crowd, looking forward to what would happen.

When Kama saw the petrified and withdrawn Shiva, he situated himself strategically. He waited patiently until Shiva's gaze would fall upon Parvati. Parvati approached Shiva and placed some flowers on the Shiva linga, which was in front of him.* Shiva noticed her, and when his eyes fell upon her, Kama shot and hit him right in the middle of his heart. Enraged that his meditation was suddenly interrupted, Shiva opened his third eye, the fiery eye of destruction, and its blazing flame burned Kama immediately into a pile of ashes. Shiva now closed his eyes again and wanted to continue his meditation. But in the brief instant that the arrow hit his heart, he had also seen how beautiful young Parvati was. And now he could not forget the image of the gazelle-like, almond-eyed young maiden; it had been burned into his heart. No matter how he tried not to, he always thought of her, and he felt a deep desire for her, a desire that burned like a fire

---

*A phallic-shaped representation of the god Shiva, which is worshipped as Shiva himself.

and could not be quenched. That is how the great love came to be, in the glow of which—thanks to Kama—the savior of the world could be begotten.

When the creatures heard that the god of sensual love had been burned to ashes, everyone became sad, especially the females. For this reason, Parvati asked her lover to give Kama life again. Shiva gave the boy his life back but was somehow unable to give him a new body. Since then, Kama is invisible. He now shoots his love arrows, but the beings he hits—be they human, animal, demon, or deity—do not know where they come from. Without a body of his own, Kama slips into the bodies of the lovers as they merge and become one, and enjoys their pleasure.

The icon of Kama is full of important symbols. He holds the bow so that he lets the arrow fly straight away from his own heart. The arrow is made of brightly colored flowers. In other words, flower messages are sent from heart to heart. Flowers are known to be the best way to express emotions. For every event that touches us, we give flowers— birthdays, baptisms, weddings, anniversaries, funerals, hospital visits, and visits to loved ones. By giving a bouquet of flowers to his beloved, a lover gives her his heart. The types of flowers he chooses, the size of the bouquet, the colors and scents, all reflect his innermost feelings. They are a message from soul to soul. This makes sense because plants are most animated in their flowering parts. The plant reveals its soul in the blossom—in the scent, color, delicate shapes, and (even measurable) heat of the flower. Until the rhythmically growing, rampant plant blooms, it is green and soul weaves around it from the outside. It is the flowers and fruits that bring the plant itself into the world of soul.

The parrot, who serves as Kama's mount, represents the playful chatter of the lovers as their souls commune with one another. Kama's companion and lover is Rati (love). She embodies his shakti, or feminine energy. She is the Indian Venus, the goddess of sexual passion. As such, she follows him on his journeys through the three worlds— the underworld, the world of the gods, and the human world. Kama is called by many names: he is Madan, "the one who intoxicates with love"; Manmatha, "the one who excites the mind"; Pradyumna, "the one who conquers everything"; Ananga, "the one without a (physical) body"; Pushoasara, "the one whose arrows are flowers"; Abhirupa, "the beautiful one"; Shringara-Yoni, "source of love" or Madhudipa, "lamp of honey." The Buddhists know him as Mara, "murderer, destroyer, the one who wounds (with his arrows)." Just as he is for the ascetic Shiva, Kama is also an unwelcome guest for Buddha and his followers. He embodies sexual desire and sensual longing, which, according to them, prevents enlightenment and nirvana.

St. Valentine's Day

On February 14, the day of Saint Valentine is celebrated as a time for love and lovers in the Western world. The custom of celebrating romantic love in the middle of February—"on the day when the birds begin their mating chatter"—has been known in Europe since the High Middle Ages (a time in which the climate was milder than today). The saying "Be my valentine" has been used in England since the time of Chaucer (fourteenth century). On that day, occasionally also known as the feast day of Saint Philomena, young people exchanged small gifts, love poems, or cards with big hearts; lots were drawn to determine who would be the valentine, with whom one might have a fleeting love affair, and divinations were made regarding future love and marriage. The poems usually began with "Roses are red, violets are blue . . ." The first young man a girl saw that day was considered a possible future lover or husband. On Valentine's Day in Europe, boys and girls cracked hazelnuts at festive social gatherings. If anyone found a nut with two seeds, then the others called out *"Philopena!"** and a kiss, a dance, or a date was due. The oracle with the hazelnut is not accidental: in the time of the ancient Celts, the hazel tree was associated with sexual potency, fertility, and the blessing of the ancestors who want to incarnate again on earth (Storl 2000, 206).

Since 1860, Valentine's Day has become a big business in Anglo-Saxon countries. Sellers of chocolate hearts, bouquets, and greeting-

*Variations on the word were used throughout Europe and Scandinavia.

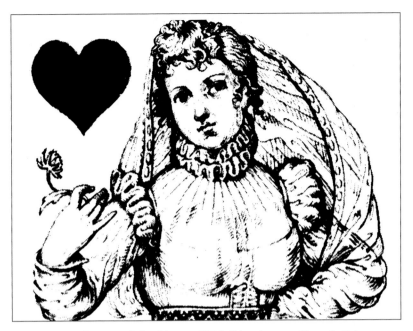

The Queen of the Heart, 1809 (Hamburger Kunsthalle)

cards enjoy brisk sales among love-hungry teens. But what does Saint Valentine, a Roman martyr from the third century, have to do with this merry feast of hearts in love? In fact, nothing! It was part of the Festival of Fools (which has become spring carnival, Mardi Gras) celebrated by the pagan Europeans when the spirits and forest sprites marched through the villages and alleyways of the cities, roughing up the people so that they themselves became wild, libidinous, and ecstatic. These spirits (people dressed up as forest gnomes and the like) turn ordered, rational everyday life upside down. By creating chaos, they open people's hearts so that they can receive new impulses, new inspirations, and even possibly a new life (children). These wild spirits, expressed in fooling around during carnival, bring fertility without which no population can survive.

Valentine's Day goes directly back to the Roman festival of fools, Lupercalia, which was celebrated on February 15, the month of Juno Februata, the goddess of feverish love (Latin *febris,* "fever"), to honor the horned god of nature, Pan or Faunus. On that day, young men sacrificed goats and a dog, smeared the blood on themselves, and cut strips out of the skin of the dead animals. Wielding these bloody strips, they ran through the alleyways, lashing at the—usually eagerly waiting—maidens, especially infertile women, so that they, too, might get pregnant that year. The festival escalated into a wild outlet for sexual excess. The young Romans drew lots with the names of the girls with whom they would play erotic games. The lovers themselves were no longer rational human individuals; they were ecstatic and possessed by the frenzy of spring and the vegetation spirits.

Of course, the Christians had problems with these lustful goings-on. For them, February was the month of cleansing. The purification of Mary, forty days after she gave birth to Jesus, fell in this month. February 14 was declared a day of misfortune and was even said to be the birth-day of the wicked Judas Iscariot! Later this day was declared as the feast of the martyr Saint Valentine, to whom various biographies were attrib-uted, such as that he, as a poor priest, healed a blind girl, or a boy crip-pled from St. Vitus's dance—wild, uncontrolled dancing done by those who are possessed by devils.* Two of his attributes are a crippled boy and a rooster. Despite all this, Valentine inevitably became the patron saint of lovers. The rooster, his attribute, is not only the announcer of the new day and expeller of the demons of the night but also a symbol of lust and the desire to mate. Later, in the Middle Ages, Saint Valentine was called upon when doing love magic or making love potions.

The Classic Heart Shape

The cards that are exchanged on Valentine's Day, in addition to the dec-larations of love, the bouquets of roses and other flowers, always depict a bright red heart. It is the classic heart shape we find everywhere: the suit of hearts on playing cards, carved into the bark of a beech tree, as a tattoo, a piece of jewelry, a shape for cookies and chocolates, balloons, pillows, on a coat-of-arms, and elsewhere. In the field of botany, one also speaks of heart-shaped leaves, such as we see on a linden tree, a

---

*St. Vitus's dance, or Syndenham's chorea, is a neurodegenerative disease.

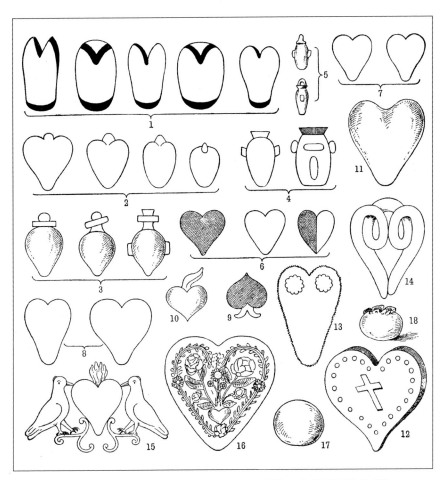

Traditional heart shapes (Hovorka and Kronfield 1909, II:65)

violet, lemon balm, grass-of-Parnassus, European birthwort, and other plants. This heart shape was often interpreted as a signature of cardiac efficacy.

Where does this idea come from, this representation of the heart with two rounded upper lobes tapering down to a point? It has little to do with the anatomical heart, which is more like a fist-shaped muscle-tube. Was it perhaps the case that the actual anatomical form was unknown? Anatomically correct representations of the heart have only existed since Vesalius, who dissected corpses in the sixteenth century. As a love salutation, the image of the heart muscle is obviously out of the question.

The mystical heart—be it the heart of Jesus or, in India, the heart of Hanuman—is always represented in the middle of the body; and yet, the anatomical organ is located in the left anterior chest. There is much speculation regarding the origin of the imaginary heart shape: some feminists claim that it is a cut-up fig or a pomegranate—symbolically the sacred heart representing the goddess's immortality—the "apple" with which Eve chose Adam as a lover (Walker 2003, 62). The ivy leaf has also been considered as a model, because in the Middle Ages ivy was a symbol of the immortal soul and fidelity in marriage.* Another interpretation traces the heart shape to mating swans and the shape when their necks bend toward each other. Swans that live on foggy waters, and have necks like snakes but are birds, have been associated in many cultures with love and longing for love. There are the enchanting swan maidens of Indo-European legends: the virgin Leda, whom Zeus, in the form of a swan, impregnates; or the Lohengrin legend. Others see in the heart shape the symmetrical curve of

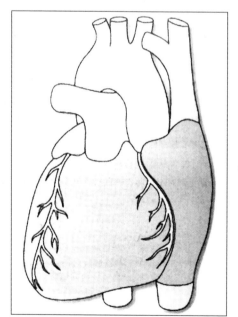

A modern heart shape

---

*Ivy (*Hedera helix*) can hardly be described as having heart-shaped leaves. The leaves of its young creeping and climbing branches are five lobed, and as the plant grows, the leaves of the older flowering, fruiting branches become egg shaped.

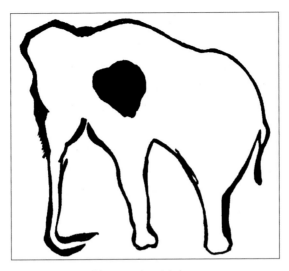

Mammoth with heart
(Paleolithic cave painting in Asturias)

the breasts or the buttocks, or the face shape of a young man with chubby cheeks and a pointed chin (Bartens 2006, 125).

And yet, the classic heart shape seems to mean even more. In the El-Pindal cave in Asturias, Spain, a rock carving of a mammoth was discovered that includes a classic heart shape that was even colored red with ocher. French archaeologist Leroi-Gourhan thinks that the image dates to the Magdalenian era, about fifteen thousand years ago. Others suspect a fake. Perhaps, however, the Valentine's heart does not directly refer to the physical hollow muscle, which pumps the blood; instead, what is represented in this form is much more the heart aura, the etheric heart, the subtle-energetic radiance of the heart chakra. Like a fountain, this energy springs from our midst and then descends, tapering off (♥). This energy movement can be simulated eurythmically with our arms, or, as is popular today, with our fingers.* This etheric heart

---

*Eurythmy is an expressive art form (like dancing) developed by Rudolf Steiner in conjunction with Marie von Sivers in the early twentieth century. Primarily a performance art, it is also used in education, especially in Waldorf schools and—as part of anthroposophic medicine—for therapeutic purposes. The word *eurhythmy* is formed from two ancient Greek words that together mean "beautiful or harmonious rhythm."

may, as the ancients said, be bright or dark; it can be tiny, withered, and hardened—so that, a Christian would claim, only the Savior's blood can make it healthy again—or it can be huge, as big as a mountain, or as big as Texas. Such a big heart, a well of love, can be found, for example, in the Indian spiritual leader Amma (Sri Mata Amritanandamayi). She embraces and presses everyone who comes to her directly to her heart. Every day she hugs thousands of people—young and old, men and women, the sick and the healthy—and gives them the feeling of having encountered their divine Self.*

Bewitchment

There are a lot of love spells centered on the heart. Clever women, and especially witches, knew (and know) how to make love spells. Through magical drinks or powders secretly administered to their victims, and by means of magical incantations, they could conquer the heart of any desired man and compel him into erotic union. They made potions with herbs such as mandrake root, lily of the valley, sea holly, and other plants under the rule of Venus; ground fingernails and pubic hair; mixing in underarm perspiration and menstrual blood; and using the hearts, testicles, limbs, blood, or semen of animals that were believed to be particularly horny, such as goats, roosters, or rabbits. Anne Boleyn is said to have ensnared the English King Henry VIII with the help of such a spell. This magic enraged the church, because monks and priests fell prey to it frequently enough—as did the occasional pope.

A candle spell is a particularly strong love spell, still known to this day. With the needle, the witch pierces the candle flame and intones: "I pierce the light like the heart that I desire." If the man so addressed proves unfaithful, it means his death (Habinger-Tuczay 1992, 251).

---

*Amma is—more than Lady Diana or Elizabeth Stuart—a veritable queen of hearts. When she embraces the people during *darshan* (Sanskrit, meaning "a vision of the truth transmitted through an enlightened person") and presses them to her breast, she seems to be in ecstasy. Why ecstasy? Through all the illusionary layers and personality masks, she sees the true essence, the divine that lies within. That is bliss for her. She embraces God in the particular form in which he stands before her. Meanwhile, she has hugged between thirty to forty million people.

A doll or an image of a man could also be so pierced in the heart. Hildegard of Bingen mentions various plants that can undo or ward off such love spells. St. John's wort (*Hypericum perforatum*), also called *Fuga daemonum* (literally meaning "flee, demon!") is particularly powerful against a love spell or voodoo in general. As the genus name *Hypericum* implies, the sunny herb can elevate the soul above any spell (Greek *hyper,* "over" + *eicōn,* "image, effigy"). Oregano, or wild marjoram (*Origanum vulgare*), wild thyme (*Thymus serpyllum*), and white heather can ward off unwanted love magic. With stinging nettle and garden valerian one could either ignite passion or disenchant an unwanted lover:

> *Baldrian, Dost und Dill,*
> *Die Hex' kann nicht wie sie will.*

> Valerian, oregano, and dill,
> The witch cannot do as she will.

Of course, love spells are still being used, consciously or unconsciously, in the present day. The products of the fashion industry, makeup, fragrances, ointments, and perfumes are all things that can secretly act on the subconscious and arouse erotic desires. And even today, these same herbs still help to protect the heart from harm.

SPIRITUS VITALIS—THE HEART AS THE PRINCIPLE OF LIFE

According to the mystics and cabalists of the sixteenth and seventeenth centuries, the soul detaches from the body at night during sleep and climbs a planetary ladder up into the sky. But the spirit of life, the *spiritus vitalis,* remains in the heart during this time. If this, too, would leave the heart, then the person would die. The ancient Egyptians said that the deceased had lost their hearts. In this sense, the heart is not only the home for the soul but also the principle of life.

In the fairy tale of Snow-White, it is said of the evil queen: "Whenever she saw Snow-White her heart would turn over in her body, she hated the girl so much. And envy and arrogance grew in her heart like a weed, taller and taller, so that day and night she no longer had any peace" (Grimm 2009, 161). She called a hunter and ordered him to take Snow-White into the woods, kill her, and bring back her liver and lungs as proof. That makes sense because the liver is often considered to be the seat of life. In other versions of the fairy tale, however, it is the heart (and liver) that the hunter is to cut out and bring to the queen.

The ethnological literature is full of examples that prove that the heart—and in any case, the blood—is considered to be the carrier of life force. Here are some examples: In the case of the Yoruba in West Africa, it was a custom of the new king to eat the heart of his deceased predecessor so that his strength would pass over to him (Frazer 1951, 343). For many peoples in Africa, the indigenous peoples of South Wales, and the Sioux of North America, the warriors occasionally ate the hearts of adversaries whom they had killed; this was done as a means to incorporate their strength as well as their courage and intelligence. The heart of the British commander Sir Charles McCarthy was consumed by the Ashanti chiefs (Gold Coast, West Africa) with this in mind, and the lower chiefs were given the dried meat, and the bones of the Englishman were kept as cult objects (Frazer 1951, 576). The same applies to hunters, who had the first right to the heart or the liver of the killed animal. Sometimes it was left to the gods and ghosts who took it in the form of a jackal, fox, or raven.

The Aztecs correctly supposed that the sun was the source of life force. It expends itself in the daily battle with the stars and other astral deities, and—in their opinion—therefore needs fresh heart's blood every day to renew its power. It was the task of the Mexican sacrificial priests to guarantee this was done. On the tops of the pyramids, they cut the hearts out of the living bodies of voluntary victims, or captured war prisoners, with razor-sharp obsidian knives and, while they were still beating, held them up to the sun as an offering.* Only thus could

---

*The Christians also know about blood sacrifice. Only in this case man is not sacrificed to a deity, but the deity is sacrificed for mankind. In the ritual of the Lord's Supper, people drink the sacred blood and eat the divine flesh.

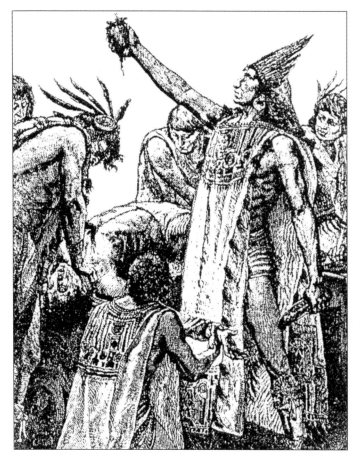

The heart belongs to the sun (Aztecan heart sacrifice).

the world be preserved, and only in this way could the field and garden fruits thrive.

The Aztec ritual—which seems cruel to us today—is not an isolated ethnological case; it is only an extreme form of the heart and blood sacrifice. In many rural and agricultural societies, a blood sacrifice of human beings or animals was believed to be necessary so that the earth could retain its power. Underlying these practices was the unwritten law that one could not take anything without giving something in return. Therefore, they sprinkled the earth with blood, or even buried body parts or hearts that had been cut into pieces in the soil. In this way, the life force passes into the soil and into the vegetables that grow there.

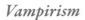

Vampirism

The recognition that the heart is the seat of the life force is also expressed in eastern European beliefs concerning vampires. The vampire is an "undead," a "revenant"—that is, a corpse that leaves its grave at night and sucks the blood of the living. By doing this, the corpse does not decay and can continue its malevolence for centuries. The vampire can be rendered harmless by sticking a spear made of thorny wood, ash tree, or precious metal (gold, silver, or gilded iron) straight through its heart, or by cutting out the latter and burning it.* As late as 1874, a few days before his death, the Romanian prince Borolajovank expressed the wish that his heart should be torn out of his corpse so that he would not have to return as a vampire like so many of his family were believed to have done. Even in the past century, in the Balkans, it occasionally occurred that a corpse suspected of sucking blood was exhumed to pierce or burn its heart (Bächtold-Stäubli 1987, III:1800). This defense against evil or alleged evil seems to have lived on even into modern times. Thus, the Nazi war criminals executed in Nuremberg allegedly had their hearts cut out, burned separately, and scattered to the winds. The same thing happened with the bear Bruno, who wandered down from the mountains in Bavaria in 2006 and was declared a dangerous bear. In a quasi-magical act, the heart was secretly removed and burned after the bear had been shot dead.†

By contrast, the hearts of those who are venerated enjoy special treatment. This was already evident with the ancient Egyptian burial rite. In preparation for embalming, all internal organs were removed; only the "immortal" heart remained in its place in the chest cavity. The Egyptians believed that the heart would speak of the deceased's former moral conduct during judgment in the other-

---

*In Indo-European mythology, the ash was regarded as a tree of the sun. The sun gods and heroes carry ash spears. The ash spear is a spear of light (Storl 2000, 280).
†*BILD-Zeitung,* June 27, 2006, page 5: "Herz des Bären heimlich verbrannt" (Heart of the Bear Secretly Burned). A bear had wandered down close to civilization and been shot. Environmentalists have succeeded in letting bears return to the wilderness in Western Europe. But it remains a struggle, as this story shows.

world (Lurker 1981, 91).* Medieval kings decreed that their hearts be taken out and buried in special places. For example, Richard the Lionheart had his heart buried in Rouen Cathedral, in Normandy, and his body in Fontevrault Abbey in Anjou. The hearts of the Bavarian Wittelsbach dynasty rest in the chapel niches by the Black Madonna of Altötting; many Habsburgs had their hearts buried in the Augustinian church in Vienna in the *Herzgruftl* (heart crypt), and the heart of Friedrich Wilhelm IV rests at the feet of his parents in the mausoleum in the castle park of Charlottenburg (Bächtold-Stäubli 1987, III:1799).

Harmful Spells, or Black Magic

In almost all cultures in which the use of harmful magic, or voodoo, is attested, there is a latent acknowledgment that the life principle is to be found in the heart. Not only in Africa or in the Caribbean but also in rural areas in Europe, wax paintings or puppets of an enemy or an unfaithful lover were—and possibly still are—made. Sometimes the heart of an animal can be found in the voodoo doll; in Europe this

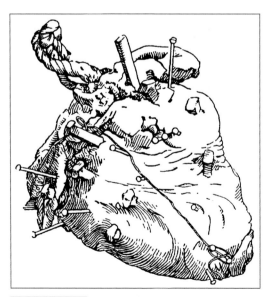

Black magic: sheep's heart with needles and nails (Pitt Rivers Museum, Oxford, England)

*Sacred, protective heart scarabs wrapped in bandages were placed on the mummies as amulets to prevent an unfavorable testimony of the heart.

was typically that of a hedgehog or a dove. If the black magician, or the witch, then pierces the doll's heart with a needle, concentrated negative, death- or disease-causing energies are directed into the opponent's vital center. The Freemasons supposedly also have a ritual in which they stab the image of a traitor in the heart with a knife or needles.

. . . .

Voodoo Death: Superstition or Reality?

Voodoo, or Vodoun, is a religion or cult of trance and ecstasy with its own deities and practices originating in West Africa and that has also gained a foothold in the Caribbean, especially in Haiti. *Voodoo,* also *Vodun, Vodoun,* and *Vodu,* from the Ewe and Fon languages, means "protective spirit." The racist sensational press has turned it into a black magic cult that primarily causes harmful magic, in particular death magic. We will stick to the standard general usage of the word and ask if there really is such a thing as a "voodoo death" and, if so, how it works. These questions were asked by physiologist and ethnopsychologist Walter B. Cannon when he was examining reports of death magic in Africa, North and South America, and Australia. This magic causes death without the use of poison or physical force.

Particularly dramatic is the bone-pointing approach used by Australian Aborigines against those who, despite being warned, repeatedly break the rules and endanger social harmony. Most of the time it is a bird's bone wrapped with a hair of the victim who is being targeted as the wrongdoer. The victim often dies within a few hours, sometimes several days after the curse, even though he or she was previously in perfectly good health. The whole tribe expects the victim's death; as far as everyone is concerned, the victim is already a dead person. Often the victim lies down, ceases to eat and drink, trembles, can neither sleep nor excrete, and dies within a short period of time.

Cannon who published the classic study "Voodoo Death" in 1942, confirmed through animal experiments the thesis that traditional death magic does indeed work. He concluded that the magically executed person is in extreme shock, like soldier's heart or shell shock, which are today known as post-traumatic stress disorder (PTSD). In the case of the shocked person, the sympathetic nervous system is activated; the muscles, including the blood vessels, contract and cramp; the pituitary gland activates the endocrine system, releasing stress hormones such as epinephrine and norepinephrine; breathing becomes shallow and fast; the digestive organs shut down; the heart pounds, and the pulse races to as many as 130 beats per minute; the victim becomes pale as the blood withdraws from the extremities, trembling and breaking out in a cold sweat; the blood-sugar level spikes. If this extreme state continues, as is the case with the victim of a death spell, the bodily functions finally collapse. After a certain amount of time, the blood pressure drops dramatically, the heart is damaged, blood plasma seeps into the body tissue, and the person dies (Cannon 1965).

· ·

Fairy tales tell of wizards and sorceresses who protect their heart, the center of their life force, by making it untraceable. A fairy tale from Holstein known as "The Man without a Heart" tells of a magician who imprisons a young woman as a maid in his house, which is secluded in the deep forest. The girl laments day and night: "You are old and could easily die, what should I do when you are dead? Here I will be, all alone in this huge forest!" The old man, who can no longer stand her wailing, sets her straight: "I cannot die. . . . Far, far from here, in a completely obscure and lonely area there is a big church, the church is well fortified with thick iron doors, and around it flows a deep, wide moat. Within the church there flies a bird; my heart is inside the bird, and as long as that bird lives, I stay alive. The bird will not die on its own, and nobody can catch it; therefore, I cannot die, and you need not worry." Finally, a young man appears, and with the help of magical animals, he finds the secret hiding place, kills the bird, and frees the maiden (Früh 1996, 114).

A Russian fairy tale recounts the story of a magician who keeps his heart hidden inside a shell, deep in a lake. A German fairy tale tells of a magician whose heart also does not live in his body but is hidden as a luminous crystal ball in the yolk of a glowing egg. The egg is in a fiery bird, which in turn is hidden in a wild aurochs. The luminous crystal ball that makes up the sorcerer's heart suggests an idea that one often encounters—namely, that the spark of the soul, the light of the soul, or the light of life that dwells in the heart. In Bavaria, a sow is slaughtered by stabbing its *Liachterl* (heart's light) (Bächtold-Stäubli 1987, III:1798). According to the old hermetic doctrine, the roots of which extend back further than classical antiquity, man is a microcosm, an image of the macrocosm. As we have already mentioned, all seven visible planets— Moon, Mercury, Venus, sun, Mars, Jupiter, and Saturn—are found in the human body in the form of seven major organs. And just as the sun shines in the center of the planets, so the heart, the microcosmic sun, radiates its ethereal light of life from the center of the body.

How Dead Is "Brain-Dead"?

The heart is the seat of life. Man has always been considered dead when his heart stopped beating. With the loss of the circulation of nourishing blood, the organs die quickly and the soul leaves the body, which then becomes a corpse. In modern times, however, a new conception of death applies. In 1968, one year after the first successful heart transplant by Prof. Christiaan Barnard in Cape Town—the patient survived eighteen days—a Harvard University commission diagnosed brain death, or irreversible coma, to be death in the legal and ethical sense. This definition, which is known as the Harvard criteria, states that a person is brain-dead "when he or she has suffered irreversible cessation of the functions of the entire brain, including the brain stem." This new concept of death (which was also written into German law in 1997) accommodates transplant medicine. Those who are brain-dead can now be exploited without reservation. Their vital organs—heart, lungs, liver, pancreas, kidneys, spleen, eyes, cartilage, and skin—can be utilized. They are now marketable commodities with an estimated value of more than $100,000 per body. Because a great many patients are waiting for donor organs, they are expensive and in short supply.* Neither the organs of bikers who died in weekend accidents nor the rather involuntary donations of executed Chinese offenders are sufficient to meet the needs of the well-to-do patients.† It follows that the commercial nature of the organ trade necessitates advertising campaigns. In a children's cinema advertisement, a young woman in a discotheque says: "This winter I gave away my heart . . . and all the other organs that could be needed for transplants." The goal of the campaign is for an organ donor card to become as ubiquitous as a driver's license in everyone's purse or wallet. The Anglican Church declared organ donation as everyone's Christian duty in 2007. June 7, 2008 was declared the Day of Organ Donation in Germany.‡ Angela Merkel appealed to the population to obtain donor cards and the popular *Stern-TV* presenter Günther Jauch held his donor card up to the camera and advised—in his function as a role model—that all good people get one, too.

One may justifiably ask: Just how dead *are* the so-called brain-dead? Their blood is warm and circulates, their hearts beat, they move spontaneously, their organs function. Until an organ is removed, the patient must be cared for, nourished, washed, and shaved. The brain-dead can have a fever. Corpses cannot. The brain-dead are even capable of reproduction. In male brain-dead persons, spontaneous erections and ejaculations occur. Pregnant brain-dead women have even given birth to healthy children and began to

---

*In the United States, the number of donor hearts needed annually is estimated at 45,000, compared with just under 3,000 donors.

†Since bikers now must wear helmets by law in many areas, the goods have become even scarcer because there are fewer brain-dead bikers. The supply from China—after all, there are about 10,000 people executed per year, from which the organs are taken—is hardly an option for hearts because the transport route to the Western industrialized countries is too far to guarantee the survival of the heart. The maximum survival time outside the body is six hours. In the meantime, the Chinese medical profession no longer (officially) advocates the use of executed persons' organs (*Deutsches Ärzteblatt* 42, 2007).

‡February 14, Valentine's Day, has also been officially designated as National Donor Day in the United States since 1998. In Canada the corresponding Green Shirt Day occurs on April 7.

produce breast milk. Spontaneous miscarriages (due to uterine contractions) are possible, as was the case with a pregnant patient with cerebral palsy in Erlangen, Germany.

When organs are removed on the operating table—or is it a slaughterhouse?—the brain-dead must be strapped down and anesthetized. The twitches, the sweating, the adrenaline rush, the increase in the pulse, and the uncontrolled (defensive) movements—in one case, a brain-dead patient clasped the hand of a frightened nurse—are dismissed as Lazarus syndrome, or spinal reflexes.

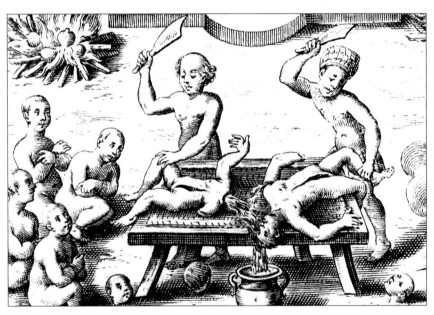

Humans on the slaughter bench, hearts burning
(cannibals as depicted by Caspar Plautius, 1621)

Apparently, the brain-dead are not really dead. It is probable—such as with people who were in a deep coma and revived, or those with near-death experiences—that there is an intact consciousness, which is independent of the brain. Coma patients often see themselves hovering outside or above their physical body and are aware of everything that happens in the room. These examples confirm the old view that it is not the brain but the heart that is the seat of life in human beings.

THE HEART AS THE
ABODE OF THE GODS

If the heart chamber is not dark and closed off, and if it is cleansed of all wickedness, then the gods—or perhaps even God himself—can come in and take up residence there. It is not so long ago that mothers or grandmothers sat down on children's beds in the evening and said a prayer with them like this:

> *Ich bin klein,*
> *Mein Herz ist rein.*
> *Soll niemand drin wohnen*
> *Als Jesus allein.*

> I am a little child,
> My heart is pure.
> Jesus alone should
> Dwell in there.

Yes, God is alive not only in the beautiful natural world outside, or far away in the starry sky, but also in our hearts. And if he is not there yet, one day he will knock on the door of the heart and ask for admission. This image of an unrecognized God who arrives as a homeless wanderer and asks for admission is older than Christianity. Odin and Balder, Zeus and Hermes, or Shiva and Parvati, appearing as wayfaring strangers, would knock on people's doors, asking for alms or a place to stay. In this way they tested people's hearts.

The theme of the divine taking up residence in the heart is a story found in many cultures. In India it is particularly prominent. The great Indian sage and guru Ramana Maharshi (1879–1950) taught the following about the process of enlightenment: When through yogic practice the kundalini serpent is awakened in the root chakra, then this primal energy shoots up through all seven centers of life, which then open like lotus blossoms blossoming in the morning sun. In the crown chakra,

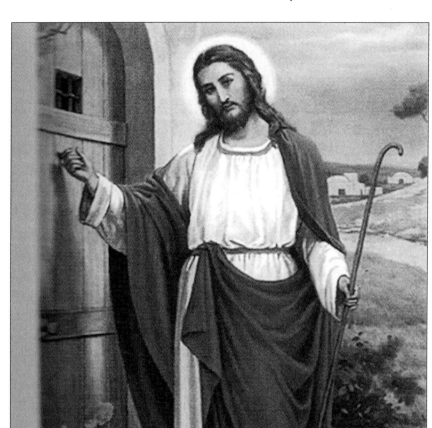

Jesus knocks on the door of the heart

the kundalini weds the spirit, the *purusha*. But after this enlightenment has taken place, the divine Self descends and resides in the middle, on the lotus throne of the heart.

Shirdi Sai Baba (1838–1918), another Indian sage, quotes the divine Self as saying: "Remember that I not only preside over your hearts but also reside therein," and "I dwell in the hearts of all beings and thus remain a witness to all acts of the beings" (Kumar 2003, 31, 75).

Krishna's followers also say that the shepherd god, the lover of souls, lives in every heart. Wherever a heart beats, in a cow, in an elephant, in a dog, in a Brahmin, and even in a "dog-eater" (an untouchable), he is present. Therefore, no living thing with a beating heart should be killed.

Hanuman's Heart

The heart is the center of what Hindus call *bhakti,* which is pure, self-less love or devotion. It is depicted in a popular icon in India, which shows Hanuman—the Europeans know him rather condescendingly as the Monkey God. He appears in monkey form because, as the legend goes, his mother was a noble monkey lady who was impregnated by the wind (spirit). Her baby was born with magical abilities. He could become as big as the largest mountain or as small as an ant; he could fly as fast as a thought. He became a master of yoga, and no one could compete with his knowledge of the scriptures. During Hanuman's lifetime, a powerful magician enchanted and enslaved the world, filling it with such a multitude of lies and deceit that joy and virtue threatened to vanish from the earth. Vishnu, the World Sustainer, and his feminine energy (*shakti*) took on human shape, as noble royal children named Sita and Rama, to save the earth.* Though they were the heirs of kings, this wicked magician had accumulated so much power that after their marriage they were not able to rule and were forced to hide deep in the forest. The magician even managed to enter the secret forest in the shape of a deer and kidnap Sita. He brought her to his distant kingdom in what is now Sri Lanka (in the story, a symbol for the far end of the world). Hanuman, who did not know for a long time who he really was and what his life's task should be, recognized their divine origin and selflessly devoted his life to them as a faithful servant and courageous warrior. Thus, the magical ape became the symbol of true *bhakta* (selfless devotion to God). Hanuman was convinced that Rama, the supreme god, can be found everywhere and in everything. When he once told his companions about this, he was laughed at as a simple fool. Then, with his mighty hands, he ripped open his own rib cage and revealed his heart: there were Rama and Sita hidden in it—a popular icon. The message: God (here in the form of Ram and Sita) lives in the heart.

---

*The story of Rama and Sita, who incarnated as king and queen, and of Hanuman, the king of monkeys, is found in the classic Indian hero epic the *Mahabharata.*

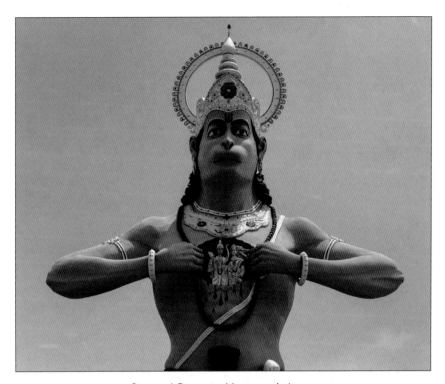

Sita and Rama in Hanuman's heart

Hanuman's virtues are heart virtues—courage, strength, wisdom, and selfless devotion. The monkey god also brings healing because he is the patron of healing herbs. Indeed, one might say that Hanuman—this inexhaustible and unstoppable faithful companion of the divine Self— is the very heart that beats within us. As Rudolf Steiner points out, the heart is the switchboard between top and bottom, inside and outside. It is the pulsating, rhythmic balance between these poles, between the respiratory and digestive processes, between organic, instinctual nature and the conscious mind. The heart, like loyal Hanuman, is half animal and half divine. Hanuman is the king of hearts. He is our heart, telling us: "From the point of view of the body, I am your servant; from the point of view of the individual soul, I am a part of you; from the point of view of the Self, I am you" (Ludvik 1994, 136–37).*

---

*From the *Mahanataka*.

Even in the Christian West there is the image of the opened breast, revealing the divine mystery. The French mystic Marguerite Marie Alacoque had such a vision in which Christ appeared to her "with five wounds, as bright as five suns." He opened his chest and let a sea of rays out of his heart shine upon her. The veneration of the Sacred Heart of Jesus in Europe reached a new peak in the seventeenth century with Marguerite Alacoque.

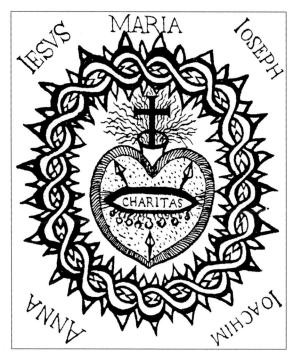

The Sacred Heart of Jesus (Marguerite Marie Alacoque, Turin, 1685)

The Dance of the Universe Takes Place in the Heart

Another Indian icon is Shiva as the King of Dancers (*Nataraja*). Shiva (Sanskrit, "the benevolent one, the gracious one") represents another conception of the original divinity that is hardly accessible to our limited minds. Shiva is often portrayed on the top of the world mountain (Mount Kailash) as a meditating yogi, from whose meditation the universe is created. In the South Indian icon, the god of gods (*mahadev*) Nataraja, dances the creation and destruction of innumerable universes into and out of being. As he is dancing, he is surrounded by a blazing wreath of fire. His wild, matted hair swirls around his head. He wears a live cobra wrapped around his neck like a scarf, a sign of his numinous remoteness. His face, however, is balanced and harmonious. One of his four hands, the upper right one, holds the hourglass-shaped drum (*damaru*), which is constantly sounding the original sound, *Om,* and thus giving rhythm to the universe, the dance of the stars, the tides of the ocean, the beating of hearts, the vibrations of the atoms. This *Om* is the vibration of the whole of creation. Opposite, in his left upper hand, he holds the fire of destruction, because everything that comes into being passes again. Another hand points to the raised left foot, suggesting lightness and ease of being. The fourth arm has an extended, open palm of the hand, signifying: "Fear not! No matter how wild the dance is, how stormy the hurricane, may peace be upon you!" The right foot of the divine dancer holds down in the dust the midget demon whose name is *Muyalaka,* "the ruthless one," a symbol of petty-mindedness, selfishness, and illusion. The dwarf is trapped in earthly heaviness and has forgotten about cosmic lightness (Storl 2004, 95).

Where does the dance of Nataraja-Shiva take place? It is the dance of the entire universe, but it takes place in the heart—in our hearts. The sages let us know: *Tat tvam asi* (Thou art that). You are not only the dwarf, trapped in the dusty world of matter, you are also Shiva, the creator and destroyer—that is the message of your heart!

Our divine Self, or God himself, lives in the heart. In a civilization in which the heart is just a pump, the divine cannot be distinguished. The intellect, bound to the cerebrum, desperately searches for logical proof of God but does not find it, or simply deceives itself. But the heart knows: it does not need proof or an ideology-based belief system.

Strict Puritans and Calvinists believed that not only the divine can rule in the heart but also that less-exalted spirits, gods, and demons can sneak in. In their black-and-white, either/or way of thinking, the heart of man is either the temple of God or the workshop of Satan. According to Calvinist theology, every person must decide for himself who should

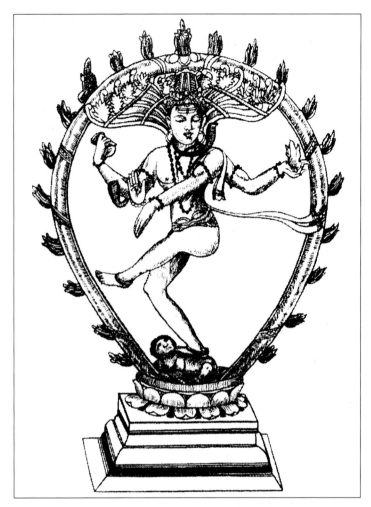

Shiva Nataraja (The Dancing King, southern Indian
icon of Shiva dancing in the heart)

live in his heart. To choose God was to choose truth and blessedness, but in this vale of earthly existence whoever made this choice probably suffered deprivation and persecution. By contrast, to choose the devil brought a life of luxury, success, power, and wealth, but also damnation for all eternity.

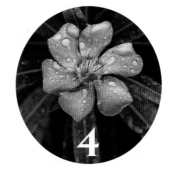

WHAT MAKES
THE HEART SICK?

*May your heart beat in harmony with the heart of the
earth,*
*May you feel that you are a part of everything that
surrounds you.*

CHEYENNE BLESSING

Herzlosigkeit ist der schlimmste Herzfehler.
(Heartlessness is the worst heart defect.)

OLD GERMAN SAYING

ANSWER I

There Have Always Been Heart Diseases—
They Were Just Not Recognized as Such

The standard answer of academic medicine is that surely before modern
times there were as many coronary diseases as there are today, they were
just not recognized as such. Science had not suffiently advanced; it lacked
the diagnostic tools, and people simply died. The understanding of the
heart and the circulatory system was confused and preempted by irrational metaphysical notions—for example, the belief that the heart could
think or perceive, that it could be enchanted, or that a psychic projection

such as God or the devil could live in the pump muscle. It was not until the sixteenth and seventeenth centuries that the tide began to turn. The earlier unscientific ideas began to crumble after 1543, when Andries von Wesel (1514–1564), known as Vesalius, dared to use sharp knives and forceps to cut open and examine the bodies of executed criminals—exposing muscles, bones, reproductive organs, veins, and hearts. His research laid the groundwork for critiquing the doctrines of the old master Galen, which up until that time had been considered infallible. Galen had taught that there were two types of vascular systems: the venous circulation originating in the liver, and the arterial circulation beginning in the heart. He also taught that the blood seeps through invisible channels from the right to the left ventricle (Porter 1999, 182). Incidentally, in the anatomi-

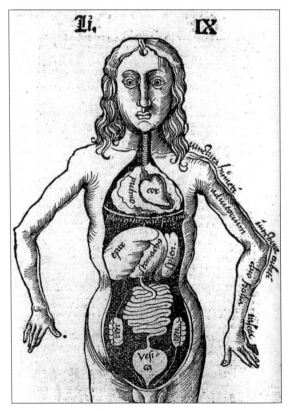

Human physiognomy according to the galenic teachings
(Gregor Reisch, *Margarita Philosophica*, Freiburg, 1503)

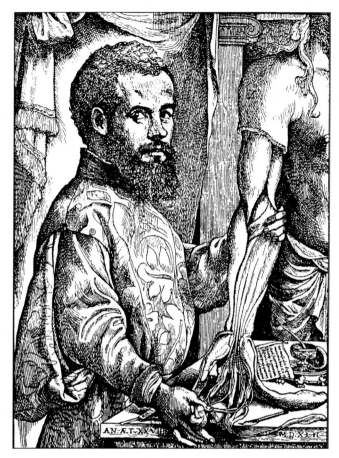

Andreas Vesalius
(*De humani corporis fabrica*, book VII, Basel, 1543)

cal dissections performed by the courageous young anatomist, monks were also present, singing liturgies so that the soul of the dissected person would not be harmed. Vesalius was, so to speak, a floodgate for the new, enlightened viewpoints, because from that point on empirical progress accumulated.

Realdo Colombo, one of Vesalius's followers, was able, through vivisection, to explain how the heartbeat functions and to demonstrate that the blood flows from the right ventricle through the lungs to the left one and that the pulmonary vein does not contain air, as Galen had believed, but instead blood, and that the blood mixes with the air in the lungs (and not in the left ventricle), where it then turns into its bright red arterial color (Porter 1999, 184).*

The elucidation of the cardiovascular system proceeded rapidly, culminating in William Harvey's (1578–1658) correct and exact description of the great blood circulatory system. It became clear by then that the blood from the heart muscle is pumped into the arteries; it does not simply seep into the body but returns to the heart as venous blood. Harvey was able to mathematically measure the amount of blood and the flow rate.† With his precise observations and experiments, he created

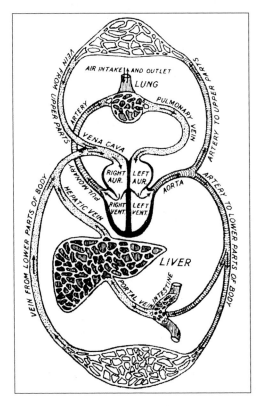

Sketch of blood circulation by William Harvey (1576–1657)

---

*Vivisection is the cutting up of a still-living animal for medical research.
†Harvey himself, however, did not see the heart as a mere mechanical pump but as an animated and animating organ. For him, man was a little cosmos, a copy of the great cosmos, the macrocosm. The heart is therefore the microcosmic sun that keeps the internal water circulation going, just as the sun circulates water for the earth by evaporation and precipitation. According to Harvey, the lungs absorb *pneuma* (life force) with the inhaled air and mix it with the blood (Heidelberger and Thiessen 1981, 96).

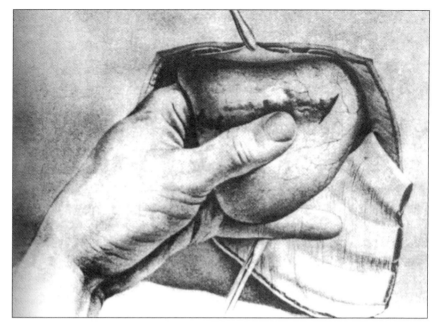

A heart in need of sewing in the hands of a surgeon
(Lejars, *Dringliche Operationen,* 1914)

the prerequisites for a mechanical understanding of the circulatory system. The development of better diagnostic options peaked in the twentieth century with the invention of electrocardiography (ECG), cardiac catheterization and phonocardiography (listening to the heart sounds), cardiac computed tomography (CT), and so on.

These advances gradually led to the new therapeutic options that are available today: implantable cardiac pacemakers (1958), heart-lung machines (1953), artificial heart valve replacement, heart transplant surgery (already in 1959, a dog received a transplanted heart), the heart bypass operation (1963), and others. In addition, the development of a whole range of drugs—blood lipid reducers and high blood pressure medication, diuretics, beta-blockers, calcium antagonists, ACE inhibitors, doxazosin, prazosin, reserpine, and so on—bring in about 3.5 billion euros annually in Germany alone, for instance. The future promises a steady development of new miracle weapons in the war against coronary heart disease. Nanotechnologists are working on tiny submarine robots that patrol and clean the blood vessels. Genetic engineers promise genetically modified mammalian tissue (which would not be rejected by the immune system) for the replacement of damaged human tissue. Genetically engineered endogenous tissue such as rtPA (recombinant tissue plasminogen activator) for the resolution of thrombosis already exists.

Recent ideas about the causes of impaired cardiovascular performance revolve around potential bacterial infections. Chlamydia and helicobacter, and possibly also viruses, could be responsible for inflammation in the inner walls of the vessels, with the result that fat and calcium deposits develop and, finally, blockage of the veins. If this suspicion is confirmed, antibiotics and vaccines may be used as therapy. Coronary diseases have always existed, but thanks to scientific progress—and provided that sufficient funds are made available—they will soon be a thing of the past. This is the conviction of academic medicine.

ANSWER 2

There Is an Increase in These Diseases
Due to Longer Life Expectancy

As recently as a century ago, life expectancy was much lower than it is today. Around 1900, men died on average at the age of forty-five and women at the age of forty-eight. From today's perspective, such a relatively short life span would not allow enough time to develop chronic heart disease. Thanks to medical progress, we live longer but suffer from age-related ailments and weaknesses, which, however, medicine is trying to get under control. Today (2021) the average life expectancy in the United States for newborn boys is 77 years and for girls 81 years. The statistics are similar in other developed countries. The global average life span is 70 years for men and 75 for women.

But such statistics should be regarded with caution. From a cultural-historical and ethnologically comparative point of view, these statements do not quite state what they seem to. They fit into the ideology of progress, the dogma that has governed the thinking of the Western world since the Enlightenment in the seventeenth and eighteenth centuries. This dogma states that humans have evolved from primitive savages to cultivated, civilized beings. The life of primitive humans must, therefore, have been "poor, nasty, brutish, and short."* We live long; they died young. Similarly, in the less developed countries, in the Third World, life expectancy is lower, but, according to this view, thanks to our developmental aid, they, too, will one day be able to share the blessings of progress.

And progress will not cease for us either. Visionaries in the medical establishment believe that hormone-replacement therapies will increase life expectancy by 30 percent and prevent age-related illnesses (Schwemmer 2000, 216). If the aging gene is discovered and eliminated, mankind can move closer to the realization of "eternal life." Vitamins and trace elements, antihypertensives, platelet-coagulation inhibitors, omega-3 fatty acids from marine fish, melatonin, DHEA supplements, growth hormones, fresh cell therapy, thymic secretions from sheep or pigs, avoidance of sunlight, and cosmetic surgery should help to counter aging, which has been declared a disease. American antiaging physicians promise a future life span of seven hundred to eight hundred years. With hormone substitution for women, testosterone, and Viagra for men, with vitamins and other pharmaceutical antiaging miracle drugs, there will be no limits to gerontological fun.†

Ivan Illich, an unflinching and courageous critic of the medical profession, already recognized years ago that despite everything, the maximum life span has not changed at all, only average life expectancy has (Blüchel 2003, 256). There were always old people—old with healthy hearts! They also existed in the Stone Age, and they still do exist among traditional indigenous societies, especially where the environment is intact and there is enough healthy food. By contrast, there have also always been times when people lived crammed together

---

*This erroneous view, first postulated by Thomas Hobbes (1588–1679), has now been thoroughly refuted in ethnological research—for example, in the work of Marshall Sahlins (1972).

†Testosterone therapies not only rejuvenate libido but also allegedly lower total cholesterol, preventing angina and heart attacks (Schwemmer 2000, 218).

in cities—in situations that favored disease carriers such as rats, mice, fleas, lice, and bedbugs—and when there was a lack of healthy food, clean drinking water, and hygiene. This was the case in late medieval feudal society, for example. It was also particularly bad in the factory cities during the Industrial Revolution. Regarding the position of the workers in the early industrial cities of England, Friedrich Engels wrote about "pale, lank, narrow-chested, hollow-eyed ghosts" who lived crammed together in human cattle stalls (quoted in Porter 1999, 399). Back then, as in the Third World today, especially infant mortality was extremely high.*

Statistics are also a tricky business. If the average mortality rate is calculated for a man who dies at the age of 100 and one who dies at birth, this produces an average mortality of 50 years. Using a similar type of analysis, one might arrive at a statistical statement according to which the average human being has one female breast and one testicle. The current birth rate and the high number of elderly people also have a favorable effect on life-expectancy statistics in modern countries, as fewer child mortality cases need to be registered and included in the calculation.

So, it is not just advanced medicine that allows us to live longer, and cardiovascular failure, cancer, and diabetes are not necessarily the results of a longer life span. Franz Konz is right when he writes:

> No—the people of the comparative groups of the previous centuries did not become very old because they lived even less naturally than we do today: most of them lived in dark tenements, in a small room, squeezed in with the whole family; the stoves were constantly emitting carbon monoxide (which had not yet been recognized as poisonous) into the rooms, and there was only flour soup, poor quality bread, and now and then a herring. Tropical fruits and fresh vegetables, light, air, sun, and sports—this was all largely unknown. The

---

*The Third World infant mortality rate is 10 to 20 times higher than that of developed countries. Four million infants die each year from diarrhea, intestinal parasites, and infections due to unsafe water and poor hygiene (Bichmann 1995, 140).

babies died in large numbers then, and tuberculosis was widespread. And this likewise flowed into the statistics that are used to elevate modern doctors. Tuberculosis was drastically reduced because the lifestyles changed—and not because of tuberculin administered by Robert Koch. (Konz 2000, 350)

Today we are healthier and live longer on average because of optimized drinking water supplies, healthier diets, and better hygiene—not because of vaccinations, preventive examinations (the periodic checkup of the bio-machine), regular medical care, or large hospitals.

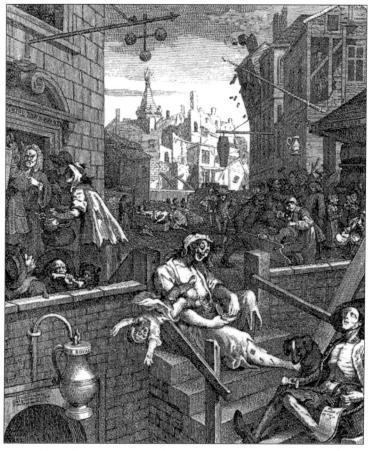

Social conditions (eighteenth-century copper engraving
by William Hogarth)

ANSWER 3
....
Denatured Lifestyle

If, compared to traditional peoples or earlier time periods, there is an increase in coronary heart disease, this most certainly also has to do with unfavorable modern lifestyles. At least, this is the view of a new generation of progressive and holistic-thinking physicians. These doctors do not simply reduce the body and the cardiovascular system to a machine. They try to view the body more as an energy field or a networked bio-cybernetic system—a complex system with internal regulatory circuits that also depend on various mental and societal factors, environmental factors, diet, and so on. Here are some things that are supposed to be good for our stressed heart pump and that will, simultaneously, make us more attractive, sexy, and fitter for a fun lifestyle.

Low-Fat Diets

We are told we eat too much fat, we are too fat (pardon, overweight!), and we have high blood fat—that it contains too much bad LDL cholesterol.

. . . .

Everyone Talks about It,
But What Exactly Is Cholesterol?

Cholesterol is a fat-like substance found in the entire organism, but especially in cell membranes, myelin sheaths, the brain, and the "cholesterol bomb"—breast milk. Cholesterol is transported in the bloodstream in molecules called lipoproteins to where it is needed in the body. There are two types of cholesterol: the good type is connected with HDL (high-density lipoprotein), and the bad type with LDL (low-density lipoprotein) (Pollmer and Warmuth 2003, 71). The good HDL takes cholesterol out of the blood, tissues, and vessel walls and returns it to the liver. There it is converted into bile acids and can be excreted in the bile via the intestine. The bad LDL transports cholesterol from the liver and intestine, where it is produced, into the body. LDL is susceptible to free radicals that oxidize it. It can form arteriosclerotic fat deposits (plaque), which mainly consist of oxidized LDL. The oxidized cholesterol can accumulate in cell walls, which, in turn, promotes the deposition of calcium. This is how LDL cholesterol turns out to be a vascular killer—or so the theory goes, at least. Animal fat contains a lot of cholesterol, but vegetable fats do not. Processed foods contain many free radicals; vegetables and foods rich in vitamins A, C, and E act as oxygen radical scavengers, or antioxidants.

So, to do something positive for our heart, we are advised to pay attention to our weight, eat less animal fat and protein, and consume more vitamin-rich raw foods, fruits, and vegetables. A diet and/or occasional fasting is also recommended. In addition, we should switch to low-fat products, from butter to margarine (which an increasing number of nutritionists now tell us is not a good idea!), from saturated animal fat to unsaturated vegetable fat. Even salt, which raises the blood pressure, should be used sparingly. High blood pressure is one of the risk factors for cardiovascular diseases. An ideal diet for the preservation of cardiovascular health was advertised a few years ago, the so-called Mediterranean diet. A study showed that Mediterranean residents suffered from heart disease much less frequently than northwestern Europeans. Health experts believed it was due to the diet—olive oil, sheep's-milk cheese, lamb, garlic, vegetables, tropical fruits, red wine, and so forth. As we shall soon see, however, these rules are not necessarily as ideal as they might seem.

Eliminating Tobacco, Coffee, and Alcohol

Smoking really is dangerous, as it narrows the arteries and arterioles. The alkaloid nicotine acts in a similar way to the stress hormone adrenaline preparing the body for fight or flight. Statistically, the risk of a heart attack is doubled if one smokes twenty cigarettes a day. Smokers taking birth control pills are particularly at risk of thrombosis (Geesing 2003, 84).

Rudolf Steiner on the Effects of Nicotine

According to Rudolf Steiner, the poison in tobacco accelerates the blood circulation and the heartbeat. This disturbs the healthy 4:1 ratio of heartbeat to respiratory rate, because the latter is not accelerated. As a result, the blood gets too little oxygen, a subconscious shortness of breath develops, and subliminal fear results. The heart beats too fast, so that its balanced relationship with other organs, such as the kidneys, is disturbed. According to Steiner, nicotine addiction is a result of the fact that humanity has neglected the spiritual aspect of life for three or four centuries. It has focused only on the material data available to the senses and the connected rational explanations. The blood, for example, which was traditionally considered to be the carrier of soul and spirit, is no longer taken into consideration as such. Tobacco—a bad habit in which many intellectuals indulge—provides a stimulus that is otherwise missing (Pelikan 1975, 1:182).

Steiner sees the heart—the "rhythmic system," as he calls it—as mediating between the head (sensory nervous system, perception and thinking) and the abdomen (metabolism, movement, and digestion). When a person loses homeostasis between these poles, the body may slip into either inflammatory or hardening (sclerotizing) reactions. The inflammatory reactions, with their heat and disintegration processes, have an affinity to digestion. The sclerotic reaction is associated with the processes of the sensory nervous system. In this head system, the dull, vegetative life processes are restricted to the benefit of consciousness. If the heart is not strong enough in its function, if the harmonious interplay of the two poles is disturbed so that the head forces become too strong, the sclerotization increases. The sensory impressions are not properly "digested." The overloaded metabolism cannot manage to eliminate all the waste and deposits. Nicotine, which is stimulating for intellectuals, pushes the balance in the direction of the hardening pole of consciousness. This can have fatal consequences, especially if physical activity is lacking due to a sedentary, intellectual lifestyle. Finally, the heart itself is included in the sclerotizing processes, and the coronary vessels harden.

Coffee has often been demonized by health fanatics. It is said to trigger everything from rheumatism to coronary disease. Too much caffeine from coffee or caffeinated soft drinks causes restlessness, insomnia, headaches, and sweating of the palms and can lead to irregular heartbeat and palpitations (Pelletier 2007, 85).

Alcohol deadens, numbs, and destroys brain cells, helping to make a dismal life bearable for many people. It is beyond doubt that excessive alcohol consumption harms the liver. But is it true that alcohol endangers the heart? It is plausible. It dilates the small blood vessels and drains the tissue. It seems to increase the blood lipid level, probably because it attacks the liver, which is responsible for the breakdown and discharge of blood lipids.

Physical Activity

According to a German adage, "Whoever rests, rusts" (*Wer rastet, rostet*). Physical inactivity is bad for the heart. Long-distance running, cycling in rough terrain, hiking, and similar physical exercise, such as jogging, mountain biking, Nordic walking, and fitness training, are recommended by experts to compensate for the lack of exercise in our modern lives. A person who works in an office, sitting in front of a monitor all day, needs such compensation. Instead of trying to relax with beer and potato chips in the evening in front of the TV, people with modern jobs should try wellness, autogenic training, yoga, and/ or dancing to relaxing music. Objective observation clearly shows that people are tense while watching TV and that it increases their blood pressure.

Reduction of Electrosmog

Electromagnetic pollution and electric fields—in particular, pulsing microwaves from cell phones, wireless telephones, microwave ovens, radio and cell phone towers, and the like—disturb the natural circuits of living organisms, including those of humans. This accumulation of electrosmog disturbs one's existential orientation, impairs the immune system, and leads to an increased release of stress hormones. It also gets to the heart. The ubiquitous electrification has us constantly under tension. We realize this when the power fails because of storm or repairs. To stay healthy, it is advisable not to sleep in the midst of electrical fields—that is, next to electrical sockets, cables, and devices that are in standby or sleep mode. Some people, who are aware of or sensitive to these kinds of influences, turn off their electicity at night; others just turn off their Wi-Fi. Many people turn off their cell phones at night, or at least keep them out of the bedroom, and some try to use them as little as possible in the daytime, too. One might also pay attention to geopathic stress lines, water veins, and the like, as they can also influence the heart and cause cardiac arrhythmia. The location of the bed can also be moved, for instance, until one finds the ideal spot. Some sensitive people enlist dowsers to help them find sources of disturbance.

Can We Live by These Rules?

All of the aforementioned recommendations are good. But who can really keep up with so much well-intended advice, and does it really offer effective protection against all of the harmful influences? Advertising, economic considerations, and external social pressure do not make it any easier. Health experts therefore try to appeal to the will of the individual. They shift the problem to a personal level. The usual message is: *You are primarily responsible for your own health.* If your heart and the circulatory system start to go on strike, it is because you haven't resisted the temptations: cigarettes; Big Macs, salty fries, and milkshakes; barbecued ribs and beer; too much coffee and sweets; or late-night raids on the fridge. You've sinned.

And the list of sins doesn't stop there. On Sunday morning you slept in instead of jogging a few miles; in the evening, you plopped down on the couch with a bag of chips or popcorn instead of going to the gym. You've shown yourself to be an unworthy body owner. Your body—and don't you ever forget this—doesn't just belong to you, it is also the property of society. If you do not follow the rules, you're ultimately antisocial. In the worst-case scenario, you might end up becoming a social-welfare case.

No one can feign ignorance: countless books, magazines, journals, TV fitness shows, weekend workshops, finger-wagging experts and physicians, friends, neighbors, and even family members constantly remind us about things that might harm us and what we should do about it. It concerns us all. Asceticism and hard work are what's needed. If we really buckle down, we are met with approval and will be rewarded with things like social success, better personal charisma, more respect, a fulfilling sex life, and better career opportunities.

Through such efforts, especially through more conscious diet and an active life, the number of deaths from coronary heart failure has decreased since the mid-1960s (Porter 1999, 586). Nevertheless, heart failure is and remains the leading cause of death in modern Western societies. The number of cardiovascular inpatient hospitalizations has even increased (Petry and Schaefer 2007, 5).

The rules for achieving greater heart health all sound reasonable. However, a closer look reveals some shortcomings and catches, which we will briefly mention here. The healthy way of life, which so many cling to so tightly, can become a big source of stress itself. And stress, as we will see in the next chapter, is one of the main causes of heart failure. For many people, the rules become the tenets of an ersatz religion, and the nutrition experts—who often contradict each other—become food populists. In line with the experts' advice, many Americans are eating less and less animal fat for fear of heart disease and more low-fat products, with the result that they do not feel full after their meals and, therefore, eat large quantities of carbohydrates (pastries, sugar), which, in turn, make them fatter and more susceptible to heart disease (Garrett 2011, 456). Meanwhile, the causal relationship between cholesterol and myocardial infarction proves to be more than questionable; it seems that lite products mainly lighten the wallet (Pollmer and Warmuth 2003, 85, 204).

High levels of LDL cholesterol are unlikely to be the cause of arteriosclerosis. Instead, both the high levels of LDL cholesterol (suggesting a blood lipid metabolism disorder) and arteriosclerosis likely have the same cause.* Fifty to sixty percent of patients with heart disease have no elevated cholesterol levels. In traditional peoples with extremely high consumption of animal fats and cholesterol, such as the Inuit, the Sami, and East African cattle herders, the incidence of coronary heart disease is much lower than one would expect according to the modern theory (Harris 1991, 36).

Meanwhile, the crusade against fats and cholesterol has reached an almost hysterical pitch. The scientific surveys that show a link between cholesterol and coronary mortality rates have significant weaknesses. There is no clear link between cholesterol and fat intake, blood cholesterol levels, and coronary heart disease. In addition, our body— especially the heart and brain—needs cholesterol. This lipoprotein maintains the integrity and fluidity of cell membranes, protects nerves and facilitates conduction of nerve impulses, and is necessary for the synthesis of sexual and stress hormones and the body's own vitamin D production. If there is insufficient cholesterol because of a low-fat diet or as a result of cholesterol-reducing pills, the body itself will produce it (Pollmer and Warmuth 2003, 75).

What really cause problems, however, are the trans fats (artificial fats) used by the food industry in foods such as margarine, chips, french fries, pastries, and various low-fat foods. Due to their non-usability and the fact that they do not stay in the digestive tract but instead spread throughout the body, these synthetic fats cause problems. They accumulate in cell walls and can cause continual micro-inflammation. They promote heart disease, cancer, and diabetes and pose a danger to unborn life by crossing the placenta and interfering with the conversion of essential fatty acids (Herrera and Ramos 2008). A Harvard study in

---

*A causality may be assumed here that does not exist. A similar false logic can be found in the current climate discussion. Higher amounts of carbon dioxide (CO_2) in the atmosphere are considered to be responsible for global warming. However, there are enough serious scientific studies to show that in past epochs the CO_2 increase has, rather, followed warming and that the cause of the periodic temperature variation on earth is not carbon dioxide but a change in solar activity. As it warms up on the planet, the oxidation processes increase and the sea—like a bowl of carbonated soda pop that is warmed up— releases more carbon dioxide (Böttiger 2008).

which the eating habits of 85,095 nurses were studied for years showed that replacing just 2 percent of energy from trans fats with unsaturated fats decreased the risk of heart disease by one-third (Willett et al. 1993).

Another question: Can we salt our food, or does salt cause the blood pressure to rise? Studies in the meantime have shown that there is no relationship between blood pressure and salt intake and that abstaining from salt can even increase the bad LDL cholesterol level.

And what about a closer look at the much-vaunted Mediterranean diet? Is Mediterranean white bread more nutritious than wholegrain bread? The Mediterranean cuisine is quite fatty, with olive oil containing high levels of saturated oils. The consumption of meat is high, the vegetables are boiled, and, in addition, southern Europe has the highest per capita alcohol consumption per day in Europe. Nutritionists Udo Pollmer and Susanne Warmuth conclude: "The Mediterranean diet is possibly better for the heart, but in a different sense than the protagonists imagined, namely, eating what tastes good, and enjoying a good drink" (Pollmer and Warmuth 2003, 222).

Speaking of alcohol, things are not so cut and dried either: many scientific studies—and not all of them funded by the alcohol lobby—confirm that people who drink alcohol regularly and in moderation live longer. This not only applies to red wine but also to white wine and beer. Half a bottle of wine or a liter of beer per day are still within the reasonable range. Teetotalers have a shorter life expectancy. Only when chronic alcoholism sets in does life expectancy fall below that of the abstainers. Moderate alcohol intake has a positive rather than negative effect on heart disease (Pollmer and Warmuth 2003, 19).

As for coffee—regular coffee drinkers, as well as fans of espresso bars or Starbucks, can relax and continue to enjoy their cup of hot coffee without a bad conscience. Long-term studies, such as those of the American Medical Association, found no connection between heart disease or high blood pressure and coffee (Willett, Stampfer, Manson et al. 1996). Decaffeinated coffee, however, appears to be not quite as healthy as claimed and may even contribute to increased cholesterol. There is also still room for the occasional pastry or slice of pie that goes along so well with coffee. After all, there is still no evidence that obese people reduce their cardiovascular disease risk by losing weight. On the contrary, mortality from heart attacks often increases after weight loss (Pollmer and Warmuth 2003, 14).

There is no doubt about one statement: exercise is good and strengthens the heart. Running long stretches at a good clip, as our hunting ancestors did in the Stone Age, boosts circulation, stimulates the lungs and the immune system's vital lymph system, purifies the tissues by triggering perspiration, and even makes people feel good because it promotes the release of euphoric hormones (dopamine) into the blood. Modern jogging was invented to prevent heart attacks. Nevertheless, it does happen occasionally that a jogger listening to the refrain "Forever Young" on his MP3 player, straining and doggedly running his 10K, drops dead near the roadside. In other words, even such healthy activities as jogging, Nordic walking, and other sports, when overdone, can become completely stressful for people in today's performance-oriented world.

ANSWER 4
Do Heart Patients Need a Psychiatrist?

In the 1980s, it became the prevailing theory that the heart health disaster was mainly the result of stress. The term *stress,* which is on everyone's lips today, is a modern word that was created as a medical term in 1936 by the physiologist Hans Seyle. It can be traced back to the English word *distress,* which, in turn, is based on the Old French *destrece,* meaning "anguish, sorrow, distress, exhaustion." Stress does not mean, as is often assumed, the kind of pressure or tension that occurs under extreme exertion from hard work, extreme sports, or fight-or-flight situations. Rather, it is a basically constant state of tension and stress that does not abate, that lasts and has no subsequent restful phase of relaxation.

Here is a typical, everyday stress scenario—described from my own personal experience:

The alarm clock mercilessly jolts me out of a dream. The guardian angel has no opportunity to kiss my soul before awakening. Although not well rested and still tired, I jump up and stumble into the bathroom to carry out the private morning cleansing rituals, which guarantee my societal suitability: I shower—confounded temperature regulation, nearly got scalded! Brushing my teeth, while grimacing in front of the mirror, I shave off the beard stubble; the aftershave burns and dominates the olfactory nerves so that no other smell has a chance. (What hunter-gatherer would obstruct his olfactory organ like this?) I spray deodorant into the armpits so as not to become a smelly distraction at work; comb my hair; squeeze into fashionably acceptable clothes. No dallying! I keep an eye on the clock. Off to the breakfast nook. The spouse is also not exactly in the cheeriest of moods. The coffee machine is percolating—nothing goes without a caffeine fix. Whole-wheat cereal, orange juice—it's supposed to be healthy. I quickly listen to the news channel: weather, traffic, time, news blurbs. One should know what is going on in the world: disaster in Uganda, wage freeze, wage increase, plane crash, peacekeeping mission. Another glance at the clock: high time! I hop into the car and join the morning commute, a potential heart attack in the middle of a traffic jam. Damn it, please let me be on time today! The boss looks like someone has gotten his goat. And what is that sneaky, backstabbing coworker Smith up to again? Dull work routine, the daily intimidations. But at least I have work. Watching the clock. Time just does not seem to pass, it moves at a snail's pace, like molasses. But at some point, it's finally time to leave. Rush hour. Traffic jam on the highway. Wiped out, I am home again. The spouse is also knackered. Check the mail: invoices, reminders from bill collectors, advertising. Quickly put something in the microwave to quench the hunger. Or should we eat at the Italian place? Crack open a beer. TV—a flood of provocative images overwhelms the soul, images that usually have hardly anything to do with anyone's soul life but are nevertheless absorbed into one's head before bedtime and need to be worked out somehow. Tense people often do not have deep or restful sleep; maybe a sleeping pill will help. And on and on it goes: the next morning, the same routine, and the day after that it starts all over again. Weekend: time to mow the lawn and deal with annoying visitors. This is what goes on, week after week. The longed-for vacation: more traffic jams, tourist hustle, whoop it up and get drunk a few times—and everything is absurdly overpriced. The new car is still on a payment plan, taxes are due, alimony, and all the compulsory insurance, and the kids need the latest clothes, otherwise they won't be "in." Is it any wonder many people feel like they are in a hamster wheel and running ever faster?

What has just been described is a typical stress scenario. One can never relax properly, let the feet dangle, slip into a daydream—or Dreamtime, as the Aboriginals in Australia describe it. Such a life has its price, and the first one is health. The animal in us, the reptilian brain, does not understand the constant tension. Who is after us? Who wants to eat us? Who wants to fight over the spoils, the territory, the female? Instead, the reaction is instinctive: the pituitary gland releases hormones into the blood, which in turn stimulate the adrenal glands to expel epinephrine (an anxiety hormone) and norepinephrine; the sympathetic nervous system is constantly in a state of arousal and keeps the body ready for fight or flight so that the muscles remain tense, the arteries constrict, blood pressure goes up, and the heartbeat accelerates. If one could relax, these reactions would go away. But the pressure somehow just remains constant.

During chronic tension, more and more inflammatory corticosteroids enter the blood, the blood pressure continues to rise, and finally the kidneys are damaged. Then small cracks occur in the overstrained arterial walls. These are sealed with cholesterol platelets and mended, forming a kind of scar tissue with cholesterol deposits. This is how calcification or arteriosclerosis begins (Pelletier 2007, 73). Over time, the blood supply of coronary blood vessels is reduced. The heart begins to starve. Cholesterol platelets can also get loose and may be carried through the bloodstream to the heart, where they clog the coronary vessels and thus trigger a shortage of oxygen. Or they can get into the brain and increase the risk of a stroke.

A counterpart to this—also from personal experience (Storl 2003, 165)—is the life on a farm, as it has been lived for centuries in the Western world, until the beginning of the twentieth century. The peasant culture—though not to the same extent as the hunter-gatherers of past cultural epochs—was completely embedded in the daily and seasonal rhythms of nature. Unlike the wild, non-sedentary hunter-gatherers, peasant life was backbreaking work, but working was like breathing: the tension was followed by relaxation, just as exhaling follows inhaling. No shrill alarm roused people from sleep. When one heard the rooster crow at dawn, one might turn over again for a bit and continue to doze until the cows mooed ever louder in the stable because it was time to milk them. Then one got up sleepily, pulled on trousers and barn boots, greeted the dog, fed the cows some fragrant hay, grabbed the milking stool, sat down under the first cow, and began milking. It sounded like music when the streams hissed into the bucket, first in high tones, then becoming duller. Cats darted around hoping for a swig of milk. The cow sent a huge quantum of warm love energy to the milker, for to her the milker was akin to her suckling calf. After feeding and milking came the breakfast the farmer's wife had cooked: porridge from the grain harvested last August; fresh milk from the morning's milking; plus cheese, bacon, and an apple from the backyard orchard. That tasted good and gave strength. But first, the farmer said the blessing for the day. And so it went on: feeding, pitching manure, caring for chickens and pigs, cattle, and horses and, depending on the season and time of day—and usually the phase of the moon, too—taking care of such work as plowing, harrowing, sowing, planting, cutting grass, making hay, harvesting potatoes, slaughtering various animals for the needs of the family, composting manure, cutting trees, splitting wood, making shingles, repairing fences, and what all else is necessary for farm life. One was never quite finished; there was always something to do. In the evening one was tired, but still awake enough for a story, a joke, or a riddle that one might sleep over: "It stands in the field, grows tall, has nine skins, bites us all." (The onion.)

Caring for animals and working with horses is not the same as working with machines. Animals have souls—one can talk to them, share feelings with them, and they understand a lot more than meets the eye. From heart to heart, one can communicate with them. Today we may know a thousand scientific facts about animal behavior, but who can still talk to them in this way?

Peasant and farm labor, for centuries the occupation of three-quarters of the population in the Western world, is varied, physically demanding; it challenges the will and the spirit. Communal festivals, which, like the work itself, were in tune with the seasons, with the pulse of the sun and the earth, were regular occurrences that gave the people a break from the hard work.

What sounds so romantic to our ears now was hard work. Muscles and joints occasionally hurt—but it was not stress like we know it today, and it was a rhythm the heart could live with very well. Farms like these are almost nonexistent today. Though the specialized agricultural production corporations that have taken their place do facilitate the operations (which are also much more large scale), it is accompanied by previously unknown stress. One exception is the Amish, a farming community in North America that has rejected technology and yet has a healthy community and economic life (Storl 2003, 31).

What is outlined here as two opposing ways of working and living was typified in the 1960s and 1970s in the work of Friedman and Rosenman on the individual human being (Rosenman et al. 1964, 15–22). The two cardiologists, who wondered why cardiovascular disease increased fivefold between 1920 and 1970, observed more from a psychological rather than a sociological perspective. They differentiated between two personality types, the stressed Type A and the more relaxed Type B, with Type A proving to be particularly susceptible to coronary disease.

The Type A is constantly running on adrenaline. This personality is a workaholic, driven, and constantly suffers from a lack of time. Commitments, deadlines, competitiveness, and ambition are what drive this type of person. The Type A often sits on the edge of the chair, as if she or he wants to jump up right away. On the highway a Type A tries to pass everyone else; there is never a minute to waste. This kind of life runs according to a program, which includes free time as well—there will even be a program for the kids. Type A personalities like to express life in numbers: how much they earn, how many laps in the swimming pool or how many kilometers they jogged, and how many deals they have made. A Type A is impatient, tense, and backstabs all competitors—but has personal aggression under control and wears a "keep smiling" mask. This constellation of behaviors makes a Type A into a candidate for heart disease. The Type A needs psychological counseling.

The Type B, on the other hand, is more relaxed and less hostile and ambitious. This type of person can relax without guilt and works because she or he enjoys working.

Friedman and Rosenman conclude that it is not so much the intake of cholesterol as psychological factors that cause biorhythms to go awry and that lead to cardiovascular disease. Therefore, heart disease is not only a somatic (physical-biological) but also a psychological problem.

ANSWER 5
....
Sociocultural Norms—The Ethnomedical View

Ethnomedicine has a different perspective on the epidemic of heart disease. It has a broader understanding of health disorders beyond seeing them as merely the result of faulty biological processes, a lack of self-discipline, or psychological programming; it also views them as cultural patterns. Every culture defines, explains, interprets, and deals with health and illness differently. That which is defined as a disease in a society is interwoven with—and arises from—the cultural environment. The perceptions that people have of physical lapses, infirmity, and suffering are culture specific. What is considered to be an illness in one culture—such as PMS, obesity, or hearing spirit voices—is not a problem or may not even exist in another culture. *Susto,* a frightful disease in which the soul leaves the body, and the person becomes sick and depressed, is a phenomenon of Latin American culture. *Amok* is a culturally specific syndrome in Polynesia, Indonesia, and Melanesia; it is characterized by apathy, followed by aggressive states of arousal. *Piblokto,* or "Arctic Hysteria," characterized by self-destructive actions— such as running naked into a blizzard—followed by a coma, is a disease of the Inuit culture. *Tarantism* was the name given to a disease that predominantly affected women in southern Italy between the fifteenth and eighteenth centuries in the sexually repressive culture of the times, and for which the tarantula bite was blamed. The symptoms were melancholia, heavy breathing, sighing, swallowing, trembling, and fainting. Exuberant dancing to arias with emphatically sexual movements was considered the only therapy option. In this sense, one can also understand heart disease as a culture-specific syndrome of modern industrial society.

The mechanistic model of a worn or malfunctioning pump may be true to some degree. The interpretation of the current heart disease epidemic as a wealth problem caused by lack of exercise, bad food habits, use of various intoxicants, and chronic stress also rings true enough. However, neither the increasingly elaborate maintenance and repair of the blood-pumping apparatus, nor the tedious adherence to rules and practices regarding lifestyle and nutrition, have prevented the existing health catastrophe. Even the steadily growing arsenal of medicines has brought no real change.

It is our culture itself that generates heart failure. It produces specific diseases, just like it creates commercial infrastructures, high-speed transport, pollution, literacy training, a money-based economy, electronic virtual worlds, digital timepieces, ways of thinking and prohibitions against other ways of thinking, and infinitely more besides. Other cultures have different visions and goals, different concepts of time, and other diseases; they construct their reality differently and have different results. The physical condition of a person is also not merely a given or dependent on individual volition; it is embedded in the cultural constructions, in the basic values and ideas of the respective society. Cultural factors shape a person from the womb: even what the mother eats, what kind of musical rhythms she moves to, when she goes to sleep and when she gets up—all of this is formative. These kinds of cultural factors will be examined in more detail in the next chapter.

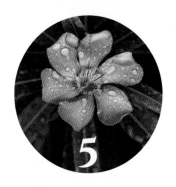

THE HEART ON THE GRINDSTONE

The clock, it shows the hour,
The sun divides the day;
But what no eye ever saw,
Is measured by the beat of our heart.

FRANZ GRILLPARZER,
MIT EINER UHR (WITH A CLOCK)

Unlearn time,
that your countenance shall not waste away,
and with your countenance, your heart!

HANS CAROSSA, *FÜHRUNG UND GELEIT*
(GUIDANCE AND COMPANIONSHIP)

TO PROPERLY UNDERSTAND SUCH A THREATENING health problem as heart disease in the Western world, ethnomedicine attempts to shed light on historical cultural contexts. This discipline asks: What differentiates our heart-threatening civilization from those more traditional societies in which heart disease is hardly an issue? One important factor is our culture-specific approach to, and our perception of, the phenomenon of time—because time is experienced and understood differently in every culture. For internationally renowned medical anthropologist Beatrix Pfleiderer, this is a key to understanding the problem (Pfleiderer, Greifeld, and Bichmann 1995, 192).

CULTURAL FACTORS: TIME PERCEPTION

We think we know what time is. Our watches and calendars measure it exactly. However, we also acknowledge that there is something like a subjectively felt kind of time. When an event is exciting and interesting, time passes quickly: "time flies." On the other hand, at work or at school, it often seems to pass slowly, sometimes even torturously so. In school we learn that time is, objectively speaking and "in reality," something other than what our irrational perceptions suggest. Time consists of a uniform ticking of time bits. These units can be measured objectively with a chronometer, such as a watch. Straight like an arrow, time shoots from an irrevocable past, through the present moment, and into a not-yet-existent future.

Within a certain time span one can take care of many tasks, do various activities, and create things. Anyone who accomplishes much is hardworking, useful, and deserves respect. Time well used means gain—as one may say, "Time is money" or "Another day, another dollar." Like a commodity, time can be saved, invested, taken, given, or even gifted to someone. Time is a precious resource, and it should be handled reasonably, managed well and rationally, preferably with schedules. Timetables are used to train students for rational time management. In the workaday world, the time allocated for work cycles and pauses is calculated exactly. Even the free time, the breaks, are increasingly organized and exactly timed. For "dreamtime" there is no time.*

Dreamtime is an ethnological term derived from the Australian Aboriginal concept known by terms such as *alcheringa, tjukurpa,* and *wangarr*. These indigenous people refer to the reality outside of time, the "inside" of the world, where the deities and creative ancestors operate, where the world of phenomena has its origin, as Dreamtime. In Dreamtime the light dreams the plants, the earth dreams the landscape, the totemic ancestors dream us. One can enter the dreams of the primordial beings. This is what the animals, the dogs, cats, and others do when they are not active, but lie idle: they dream themselves into Dreamtime. Children, healing powers, and insights come from Dreamtime. In modern civilization, Dreamtime journeys and meditations are replaced by the images of television.

On the other hand, we can waste or even "kill" this precious commodity. In the Bible Belt, where I grew up, wasting time was considered a sin. We youngsters were warned that "idle hands are the devil's workshop!" Playing cards, going to the movies, or just hanging around was frowned upon. Mexicans, punks, Native Americans, and Blacks were considered lazy because they did not use their time constructively and productively. That made them less valuable. They preferred to play music, relax on rocking chairs on the veranda, or loiter around gas stations, smoking and daydreaming, instead of cleaning up, mowing the lawn, or having a more demanding job. Unemployment was no excuse for idleness. After the civil rights legislation in the late 1960s, it was considered unacceptable to judge others in this derogatory way; such overt racist and ethnocentric prejudices are no longer tolerated. What has remained, however, is the basic understanding that time should be used productively—this view has not changed. Therefore, various initiatives have been made to develop, educate, and better integrate these underprivileged minorities, whose time paradigm does not conform to the norm, so that they, too, can learn how to deal with the precious commodity, time, efficiently.

Where time is money, there is compulsion to perform. Because we never have enough time, we are rushed by the clock; workaholics are the result. We cannot afford to waste time, because we are under pressure. In this situation, certain specific drugs are offered to help keep up physically and mentally. Coffee, cola, energy drinks, maté tea, guarana, Mormon tea (ephedra), and other energy drinks containing caffeine, theophylline, or theobromine, along with various amphetamine-based uppers that stimulate the cerebrum and, like stress hormones, often increase the heart rate, support our cultural focus.* All of these are readily available and socially approved drugs. By contrast, substances that are still generally illegal and punished by the drug police include mind-expanding, dream-provoking drugs such as marijuana, opium,

---

*Although some psychoactive stimulatants such as cocaine remain illegal, they are, nonetheless, actively used in the creative circles of society, in business, and in the arts.

peyote, psychedelic mushrooms (*psilocybe, panaeolus, stropharia,* etc.), ayahuasca, and the like. These can change our perception of time and dampen the incessant high-speed pace of modern life. They seduce us to dream, create visions, expand the limits of the ego, broaden awareness, challenge socially organized time, and might even lead to our abandoning the performance system altogether.

As a counterweight to the socially acceptable stimulants that are consumed daily, alcohol—another legal, socially acceptable substance—seems somehow necessary. Many people try to wind down and relax in the evenings with a much-anticipated glass of wine, a cold beer, cocktails, or sedatives (benzodiazepine tranquilizers, antidepressants), which are enjoyed as a means to slow things down and relieve tension. Western technological culture and its inherent concept of time is not beneficial to living organisms. The natural biorhythm, especially the natural rhythm of the heart, is overpowered; the pump in the chest begins to falter. This civilization has strapped people into a "heart-attack machine," as Bob Dylan formulated it in one of his songs, and fatally exhausts them.* Every second disease in the Western world is a cardiovascular disease. It is no surprise.

In Harmony with Cosmic Rhythms

It does not even occur to us modern people that there are concepts of time other than our interchangeable, linear, quantitatively measurable one. However, anthropologists encounter quite a variety of different ways in which time is understood in non-Western societies. They usually come to realize that not only our concept of time but also our actual experience of time are cultural constructs. The Pueblo Indians, for example, have not only one time, but each creature has its own time: the corn in its growth, the arrow in its flight, the river in its flow, a person in its life. The ancient Celts visualized time spatially. The seasons of the year, such as springtime, were seen as a room into which one enters

---

*"Desolation Row" on the album *Highway 61 Revisited* (1965): "Then they bring them to the factory / Where the heart-attack machine / Is strapped across their shoulders."

and leaves when the next season, such as summer, stands at the door. All beings—whether gods, humans, or other creatures—go from one time space (be it a day, a month, a year, or a lifetime) to another. Some Native American cultures believe that time is a kind of energy that can run down and become weak and that it is necessary for humans to rejuvenate it through rituals and sacrifices. This was partly the background of the Aztec heart-sacrifice rituals.

For the Australian Aborigines, what we call past, present, and future coexist in Dreamtime. The so-called past has not disappeared, and the future has not yet appeared; nonetheless, they fully exist, as does the present. The original Dreamtime is visualized in their rituals, and thus the creation—the dream of the ancestors—is preserved.

In the ancient Iranian and Semitic cultures, time, accelerating more and more, flows from a beginning (Alpha point) to an end (Omega point, Apocalypse). It flows like water into a pitcher until time is "filled." For other cultures, time might run backward and forward like a weaver's shuttle, flitting back and forth and weaving the carpet of reality. For most non-industrialized and traditional cultures, however, as was the case among the indigenous peoples of Europe, starting with the megalith builders, time moves in an eternal cycle, like a wheel. What has passed will return: day after night, summer after winter, full moon after new moon, the periodic reappearance of the Dog Star (Sirius) on the horizon, the fresh seedling from the seed of last year's plant, a new birth after death. Whoever wishes to know the future must submerge the mind deep into the past and see that everything returns cyclically. The time on earth—the vegetation periods; the seasonal migration of the buffalo, the salmon, the swallows—is in harmony with cosmic cycles, with the sun, the moon, and the planets. And our human daily experience, as well as a whole life's experience of time, is similar: our childhood, adolescence, maturity, old age, death, and rebirth. Whoever is in harmony and lives with the rhythms of nature—or as the Sioux say, "with the heartbeat of Mother Earth"—will have a healthy heart.

For the ancient Aryans (from Sanskrit *arya,* "noble, person of high rank")—as the Vedic Indians called themselves—the sun (Aditya,

Savitr, Surya) gives the universe the rhythm of life.* The *Aum* (*Om*), the creative primal sound, the vibration that sustains and strengthens everything, bursts out of the sun's light. This rhythm is the all-enlivening cosmic order, *ṛta* (*rita*) or *ṛtam* (*ritam*). Our words *rite* and *ritual* (from Latin *ritus*, "rite, custom," and *ritualis*, "relating to religious rites") are related to this term. The *ritam*, the heartbeat of the cosmos, determines the times of the day (morning, noon, evening, midnight), the seasons (spring, summer, autumn, and winter), the moon's phases, and the harmonious dance of the stars and planets. The gods (*devas*) live in harmony with the *ritam*, but the demons (*asuras*) do not. In the small universe of the human body, it is the heart that beats this pulse of life. Both rhythms—that of the big and the small world—are in harmony. Or at least they should be, otherwise *anrita* (falsehood) rules. In this case everything becomes arrhythmic, dissonant, wrong, chaotic, sick, and falls to ruin, delusion, and suffers under illusion.

The Aryans, as well as other Indo-European societies, consequently sought to live in harmonious union by following daily rituals from the sun salutation to the evening devotion; performing seasonal ceremonies, sacrificial feasts, and periodic pilgrimages; and observing the four successive stages of human life, called *Asramas* in Sanksrit: in the beginning of life, as a learning, serving, and chaste youth (*Brahmacharya*); during the second stage, as a steward in the enjoyment of sensual (also sexual) pleasures and with familial obligations (*Grihastha*); after raising a family, as a forest recluse, who—usually along with the spouse—withdraws from everyday life and reflects on the divine foundation of Being by listening to the wise and studying the scriptures (*Vanaprastha*); and finally as a homeless wanderer (*Sannyasa*) on the way to the ancestors. Later, the term *dharma* (from the Sanskrit root *dhṛ-*, "to hold, support") replaced the word *rita*. *Dharma,* meaning "the right way, in

---

*This ethnological-linguistic term for the Indo-Iranian branch of the Indo-European language family was unfortunately abused by racists in the nineteenth and twentieth centuries in the service of a misanthropic ideology. Nevertheless, the term remains the correct name for the immigrants settling in the Indus Valley and who have left us the Vedas and were the main source of Hindu culture.

tune with the truth," is that which one can trust in to carry one safely through life. The Indo-European tribes that populated Europe had similar notions of time, of how to live in the world, and of duty.

The Time Machine

How and when did this harmony, this *ritam,* go astray so that the people in the Western world came into such distress? The ideas and habits regarding time and reality in which we are trapped are not inherent. They are a cultural construct—a historically grown, morphogenetic field. The Celts and other ancient European peoples tried to live in harmony with the rhythms of living nature in much the same way as their distant relatives, the Indian Aryans, did. They also knew about the interwovenness of natural cycles and dreamtime, of the otherworld, which is the background and origin of the world of appearances. In this otherworld, where one can meet spirit beings, elves and demons, gods and giants, time passes differently: it goes slower, it approaches eternity. In places of power, on sacred mountain heights and at springs, where the Christian missionaries later built their churches or monasteries, this eternity shimmered through the temporal veil.

Not only geographically, where one realm shifts to another (for example, at the sea shore or the edge of the forest), but also when one time period passes to another (such as at solstice or equinox or dawn and dusk), the threshold to the otherworld can be crossed easily; during such times magical realms can open. These are the magical days when one season moves into another or the moon phases change and also includes the witching hours of noon and midnight. It was the old belief that those who did not have the wisdom of a Druid or the foresight of a clairvoyant could stumble upon dreamtime at such interim times and succumb to a kind of spell: they could be enchanted by elves or dwarves and be unable to find the way back into everyday life. What seemed like a few moments to such a spellbound (or even crazy) person was often a period of months or years in the everyday world.

In ancient cultures, care was taken to ensure that the relationship with the dreamlike otherworld and its inhabitants was kept in even balance. Only in this way could the individual—as well as the household, the clan, and the whole village—stay healthy. As humans, we belong not only in the matter or material of everyday life, but we also have a place in eternity and the kingdom of the spirits. And the heart, the center of our being, belongs to *both* sides: it receives impulses from above and below; it mediates between consciousness and the unconscious, between the here and the beyond, between temporality and eternity. A culture like our modern one—which assumes the right to deny eternity and the otherworld, or explains it away as irrational and subjective symbolism, or reduces it to a matter of brain metabolism and neurotransmitters—becomes unbalanced, loses track of the rhythmic pendulum, and ends up like a listing ship.

The ancient Greeks, to whom we owe many elements of our culture, had two terms for time: *chronos* and *kairos*. Chronos is measurable, interchangeable, expiring, linear time. Chronos is the name of the god who separated the primordial unity: he squeezed himself between his heavenly father, Uranus, and the earth mother Gaia, who were embracing each other in intimate, blissful union. He levered with all his might and pushed them apart; this created the space for himself and his siblings. Now that heaven and earth were divided, space and time emerged. The drama of creation could begin. Chronos himself, as the god of time, devoured the children given to him by his sister and wife, Rhea. Time devours everything.* Etymologically, *chronos* means "to crush; to wear, erode." Chronos appears as a miller, just as his Roman counterpart, Saturn, is seen as a reaper with a scythe and a sack of grain (Huxley 1976, 199).

Kairos, on the other hand, is the unique time, the right time—the auspicious moment. He is portrayed as a winged youth. Always on the move, he flies from now to now, as free as the wind. Wherever he appears, voracious Chronos, devouring his own children, must pause for a moment. Kairos is time in the sense of Ecclesiastes (3:1–8) in the Old Testament:

---

*In Indian mythology, Kali (the Black One) is all-devouring time that annihilates every manifestation, even that of the supreme God.

To every thing there is a season, and a time to every purpose
    under the heaven:
A time to be born and a time to die;
A time to plant, and a time to pluck up that which is planted;
A time to kill, and a time to heal; a time to break down,
    and a time to build up;
A time to weep, and a time to laugh; a time to mourn, and a
    time to dance;
A time to cast away stones, and a time to gather stones together;
    a time to embrace, and a time to refrain from embracing;
A time to get, and a time to lose; a time to keep, and a time
    to cast away;
A time to rend, and a time to sew; a time to keep silence,
    and a time to speak;
A time to love, and a time to hate; a time of war and a time
    of peace.

This time, which is called Kairos, is children's time, the time of lovers, magical time. In America it is often called Indian time. When the Native Americans hold a ceremony, they never look at the clock but instead wait until the time is right, until the spirits are all there. Sometimes this can take hours, sometimes days. In India one can also encounter this concept of time. A typical concert with tabla and sitar, as one might attend in a big city like Delhi, is announced for a certain time; but when it starts, no one can really say. People come and go, children run around amid the assembled guests, the musicians tune their instruments for what seems like an eternity, and, gradually, before one knows it, everything falls into place and the concert is in full swing. It stops when the inspiring spirits, the goddess, or the Gandharvas, the invisible heavenly singers, have dispersed once more.* And these celestial beings do not keep to earthly clock time.

---

*Gandharvas are enchantingly beautiful, angel-like deities who, with their music and songs, intoxicate even the gods. They know about love magic and medicine. They prepare the intoxicating soma, the potion of immortality, for the gods. Their companions are the spell-binding heavenly nymphs, the Apsarasas. Flowers and the fragrance of incense attract them.

The Europeans of old also knew about the "right time," a time of inspired fortune, a favorable opportunity, as *time* (Old Norse *tími,* "right time, fortune"; Old English *tíma,* "opportune, lucky time").* This concept has recently returned to our language as "timing" or "good timing." The related word *tide,* which originally also meant "time" (Old English *tíd,* "time, period, era") came to refer to the moon-bound ocean tides and their ebb and flow. According to this view, time is not something you can lose or run out of, something that runs away and must be chased after constantly, but time is a calm and regularly breathing space, a coming and going like the breath, the heartbeat, or the tides (Legros 2003, 31).

It seems that in our modern society, with its chronological time, we have forgotten the magical time, the dreamtime, the happy, auspicious time, the Kairos. Our heart, our soul, needs this Kairos, otherwise it will be crushed by Chronos and will deteriorate.

It is in this sense that the wise words of Smohalla, a shaman of the Wanapum tribe, are to be understood. He told the missionaries: "Our young men should never work. Men who work cannot dream and wisdom comes to us in dreams!" (McLuhan 1972, 56). The wandering ascetics known as sadhus in India also say that they never work so that they can constantly meditate on the divine and help it manifest on earth. The etymology of the modern German word *Arbeit* is revealing: in ancient times it connoted "hardship, bondage." The earlier word, which can be reconstructed as Proto-Germanic **arbejidiz,* in turn derives the Indo-European **orbho-s,* "orphan," and the Germanic **arb-ej-o,* meaning "I am orphaned, and a poor child forced to do hard labor" (Pfeifer 1995, 55).† This kind of work is the opposite of joyful activity in harmony with life. As the Taoists say, true social order does not emerge until people can do what they like doing, what comes natural to

---

*Luck (German *Glück,* Middle High German *gelücke,* Middle Low German *gelükke,* Old Frisian *lukk*) connotes an "accidental, surprising coincidence of favorable circumstances," so to say, a favorable gap in the flow of fate.

†The asterisks in front of words such as **arbejidiz* indicate that they are reconstructions based on historical linguistics.

them, when they follow their own nature (*tao*) and are not under the duress of an external force (Watts 1975, 77).

MILLS AND CHRONOMETERS

And now, back to the earlier question: When and how did we lose Kairos, dreamtime, the sacred, auspicious time that is in harmony with the cosmos? When did organic, rhythmic time—which resembled inhaling and exhaling, the ebb and flow, tensing and relaxing—become a merciless, monotonous, mechanical beat? It did not happen overnight but rather gradually and imperceptibly. Already with the Romans the months and the weeks were no longer synchronous with the change of the moon from new moon to full moon, as still was the case with the Celtic and Germanic tribes in the north. When the religion of the Christian God came to the north, the priests and monks—the "development aid workers" of the day—tried to educate the new converts to follow a stricter order of life; it is not nature itself that should provide the impulses and the right times for working, eating, resting, and celebrating, they preached. Bell towers were built everywhere on monasteries, chapels, and churches, and time was divided by bells. The chime of the bell announced the times of prayer, or "hours" (Latin *hora*, "hour," plural *horae*, "time"; the *horae* were originally goddesses of changing time, the daughters of the divine king Jupiter and the goddess of order, Themis).

The monastic day according to the Benedictine Rule consisted of eight main times of prayer:

Lauds (3:00 a.m.): the first cock's crow for the pious, the first prayer of the day; the time when most people die.

Prime (6:00 a.m.): work begins, around sunrise.

Terce (9:00 a.m.): a short break at midmorning, which is still known in Europe as snack time, or time for a second and bigger breakfast.

Sext (12:00): lunch break, when the sun is at its zenith.

Nones (3:00 p.m.): midafternoon prayer, work break, still observed as tea time.

Vespers (6:00 p.m.): when the day's work is done, evening prayers, dinner, time for contemplation and preparing for sleep.

Compline (9:00 p.m.): time of night prayer, bedtime.

Matins (midnight): midnight prayer.

The canonical hours made for a quite rigid time corset, but in a sense, they were still adapted to the natural rhythm. These were not yet standardized hours of equal length that tick away like a mechanical clock. The medieval monks, who had to say their prayers at the right time and ring the bells, divided the day into daytime and nighttime hours, which began at sunrise and sunset. These hours were determined according to the sun, according to the seasonal change of the sunrises and sunsets on the horizon. In the summer the daylight hours were thus longer than the night hours, and after the autumnal equinox, the hours of the day became shorter; the night hours became longer as the winter solstice (Christmas) approached. Conversely, the daylight hours grew steadily longer the closer it got to the summer solstice (St. John's Eve, June 24) (Storl 2004b, 184).

The day was like a wheel with eight spokes. In this it resembled the day wheel of the Celts, which likewise contained eight periods, and as such was a small copy of the great yearly wheel with its eight annual festivals.* As with the Celts, for the Christian monks each period had a different spiritual quality; every hour had its angel, just as each day had its patron saint and was influenced by the character of the saint.

---

*The eight-spoked Celtic wheel of the year, the roots of which lie with the megalith builders, and which at the same time represented the spinning wheel of the Great Goddess, on which were spun the threads of the fate of the world, contains: (1) the season of the winter solstice (now the twelve days of Christmas that begin on December 24); (2) Imbolc, or the full moon closest to Groundhog Day; (3) the spring equinox; (4) the full moon in May; (5) the summer solstice; (6) Lugnasad, the August full moon; (7) the autumnal equinox; and (8) Samhain, the November full moon (Storl 2000, 144).

For the Celts, the evening or eve was a sacred time. After the sun had set and the swallow flight was replaced by the whirring of bats, work stopped, and people directed their spirits toward the gods.* The Christians continued with this practice. There was even a Christian patron of the eve, Saint Notburga. Legend has it that during the harvest a farmer tried to force a young maiden to keep on with cutting the grain in the field after the evening prayers (vespers). Instead of continuing to work, she simply hung her sickle on the last ray of sunlight and went to the evening devotion. Seeing this, the farmer realized she was a saint. There is much to suggest that this girl is a christianized form of a Celtic goddess: it is said that a white doe nourished her with its milk; that snakes brought her healing herbs; and that at her funeral, two white, flower-adorned bulls pulled her hearse.

Clockworks

From the thirteenth century onward, sweating monks who pulled the belfry ropes to ring in the time of day were increasingly replaced by mechanical cogwheel-driven clocks with round dials. An attempt was made to standardize and normalize the hours. These mechanisms were driven by weights and spring tension. The tower clock had brought the planetary sky down to earth. One no longer had to look up to heaven, to the sun and the moon, to know the hour, "the stand of the sun" (Old High German *stunta,* "state, time"; modern German *die Stunde*). We hardly realize it today, but the clock is an image of the cosmos: The dial with the twelve numbers represents the fixed stars, or the twelve regions of the zodiac. The first number, one, takes the place of the ram, Aries, the head of the macroanthropos (the cosmic human); the number two stands for Taurus, the bull; three is for Gemini, the twins; and so on, down to twelve, Pisces, the fish, that

---

*In the cycle of the year, the seasonal festival that corresponded to the sacred evening was Samhain, which fell in the foggy month of November. At that time, when the dead were remembered, the year came to an end for the Celts: the work in the fields came to a rest, and herbs could no longer be gathered—they were now *pucca* (taboo) because they belonged to the spirits, the pucks.

represents the feet of the macrocosmic giant.* The movement of the clock hands is analogous to the planets passing along the solar ecliptic through the twelve zodiacal regions. The sun, which—seen from the earth—passes through the entire zodiac in twelve months, was placed as the hour hand on the tower clock. The moon, which completes the same circle twelve times over the year, became the minute hand. In the first tower clocks even the other planets, such as Mars, Jupiter, or Saturn, were considered but soon abandoned. The mechanical movements were notoriously inaccurate, they had to be continually reset according to the course of the sun.

The clock—the abstracted, cosmic rhythm brought down and banished to earth—is at the beginning of mechanistic thought. With the advent of these mechanical clockworks, the ecclesiastical-sacral monopoly on controlling time began to lose ground to the rising class of the urban bourgeoisie and merchants. This class was more concerned with earthly activities, anyway, than any kind of heavenly metaphysics. Clocks now adorned not only churches but also city gates and town hall towers.

The mechanical clock radically changed the worldview of European citizens. The universe was suddenly seen as a gigantic clockwork, as a machine that God—the Great Engineer—had designed. He was the cosmic watchmaker who had built it and wound it up and then retired after the work was done. Now it keeps ticking automatically. It will tick until it runs out of energy, and that will be the end of the world.

The great notion inspired by the clock was the idea that Creation works according to mechanical-mathematical laws, which came to be called the laws of nature. Now it became the task of the human mind to comprehend the thoughts of the divine watchmaker by exploring the laws of nature. The resulting "true and objective" knowledge

---

*The macroanthropos is the cosmic primordial man, Adam Kadmon, spread out in the zodiac, with each of the twelve signs of the zodiac being part of his body: head = Aries; neck = Taurus; shoulders = Gemini; upper chest = Cancer; heart region = Leo; belly = Virgo; kidney region = Libra; sex = Scorpio; leg = Sagittarius; knee = Capricorn; calf = Aquarius; and feet = Pisces. The seven wandering stars (planets) were thought of as the seven major organs of the great giant: moon = brain; Mercury = lungs; Venus = kidneys ; sun = heart ; Mars = bile; Jupiter = liver; and Saturn = spleen.

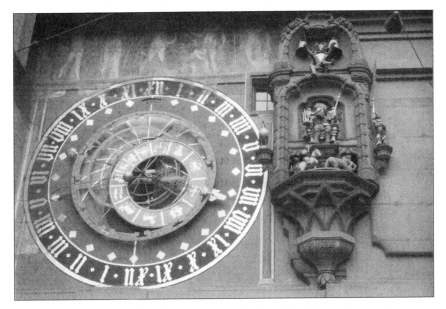

The Zytglogge medieval tower clock in the city of Bern, Switzerland

would allow for technologizing, rationalizing, and transforming human society, the working world, and indeed the whole of existence. It was no longer necessary to rely on supernatural miracles, the help of the saints, and the influences of the planetary gods and angels to explain the world. The soul of the world and the spirits in nature had served their time. God himself was no longer immanent in Creation. He had detached himself from it as deus ex machina, and he does not perform miracles—as the common folk had always believed—for these would contradict the laws of nature. Neither he, nor the angels, nor other gods bear the heavenly bodies in their hands and keep them on their course. Instead there are mechanical, mathematically calculable forces—gravity, centripetal momentum, and the like—that are responsible for this. Just like in a clockwork. Animal organisms likewise function in this way; they, too, are wound-up watches, machines, automatons. And although they might be incredibly complicated, people are machines as well. In contrast to animals, they nevertheless possess a soul, because they are in contact with the divine spirit, the Great Engineer. The connection to God takes place via the brain or, more precisely, via the pineal gland.

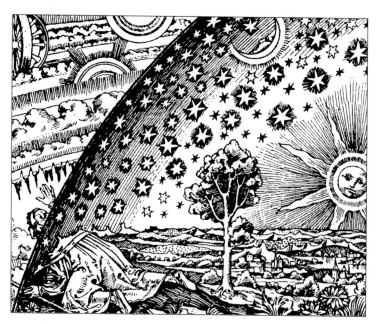

A wayfarer puts his head through the heavenly spheres
at the end of the world and sees the mechanical nature
of the universe (woodcut from Camille Flammarion,
L'atmosphère: Météorologie populaire, Paris, 1888)

That is what René Descartes ("I think, therefore I am!") believed. God no longer dwells in the heart—the organ is only a mechanical pump, after all—but has withdrawn to distant spheres, though he can be reached via the head, or rather through logical thinking.

When the heart became a pump, this was also bad for the heart's virtues, such as mercy, compassion, and sympathy. When the animals, these intricate robots, screamed and their bodies writhed in pain during vivisection, that was not an expression of suffering, it was more like squeaking of unoiled wheels or the whistling of the bellows.* Descartes

---

*This ideological de-souling of nature, especially of animals, as well as a brutal humanism that subordinates all other creatures to man, has provided legitimation for the animal experiments carried out to date. Every year, more than 100,000,000 vertebrates, from monkeys to mice, die in experimental laboratories worldwide—70 million of these deaths occur in the U.S., 11 million in Europe, and 10 million in Japan. The number is currently increasing due to genetic-engineering experiments. How can any kind of healing for human beings come from the suffering and torment of our fellow creatures?

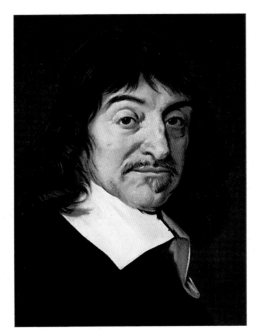

René Descartes

himself used vivisection to study the pumping mechanism of the heart: "If you slice off the pointed end of the heart in a live dog, and insert a finger into one of the cavities, you will feel unmistakably that every time the heart gets shorter, it presses the finger, and every time it gets longer it stops pressing it" (quoted in Sheldrake 1994, 53).

The clocks that provided the theoretical model for the modern age became increasingly smaller and more precise, and further detached from their cosmic prototype. The pendulum clock was invented in the sixteenth century. In the eighteenth century, elegant cabinet clocks, or grandfather clocks, became a fixture in manor houses and wealthy homes. The constant tick-tock of the pendulum clock is reminiscent of the heartbeat. Psychologically, this rhythm is so reassuring that today there are still many watches—and especially alarm clocks, ticking away on nightstands—which emit this sound effect although they would work just as well without it. Incidentally, before most timepieces were digital, it was common to hear reports that a clock stopped ticking in the moment of its owner's death.

After the wall clock came the grandfather clock, and, at the same time, the wind-up pocket watch—a timepiece as well as an article of jewelry—found its way into the waistcoat. In the twentieth century, the timepiece became attached to the person in the form of a wristwatch. In the quartz clock, a quartz crystal is inserted as a pulse regulator in the battery-operated circuit. The quartz crystal, which vibrates at 32,768 oscillations per second, enables an accuracy that can only deviate by one second over the course of thirty years. Vibrating ammonia molecules or the cesium atom are other precise pulse regulators.

Today it is no longer the sun's path that determines time for us but rather an atomic, electronic dimension that exists beyond our sensory perception. Human consciousness has descended, as it were, from the stars into the submaterial world. With the digital timepieces and cell phones we carry around, the round dial has completely disappeared; electronic numbers flicker on the display that show seconds and fractions of seconds. Who knows, perhaps we will soon be getting implanted chips that will determine our time. We no longer look to the sun, to the heart of the macrocosm—and besides, it is supposed to cause cancer. And thus we lose the final connection to the rhythms that provided the vital impulse to our existence and evolution on earth over millions of years. For the organism, for the animal in us, this release from the cosmic heartbeat means a loss of security and well-being. Unnatural rhythms lead to tension and stress. In a more profound sense, this also means a detachment from the inherent spirituality of inner and outer nature, as well as a distancing from the traditional virtues of the heart.

Millwheels

In the twelfth and thirteenth centuries, while Europeans began to place timekeeping devices on the towers of their churches and town halls, they also began to build mills: windmills and watermills for grinding grain, and then sawmills, fulling mills, and foot-powered treadmills that moved cranes and set pulleys into motion. These wind- or water-powered cogwheel machines were increasingly used to drive pumps in

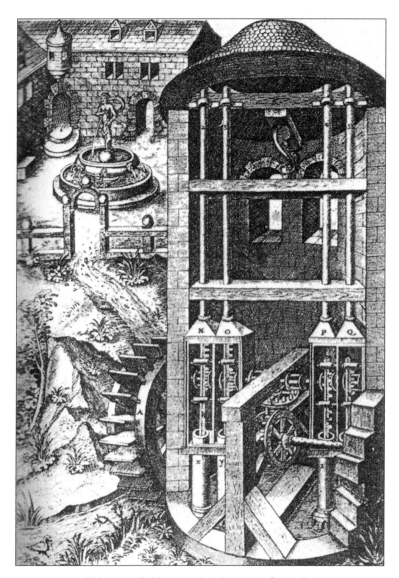

Water mill (drawing by Agostino Ramelli,
Le diverse ed artificiose machine, Paris, 1588)

mines, or to pump out marshes and fens. The power of force-multiplying devices had been discovered.

Since the Stone Age, seeds and grains had been crushed with pounding stones and mortars and pestles and ground into flour. Even in the early Middle Ages, as had been the case among the Germanic peoples and the Celts, every farmyard ground its own grain, using hand mills. But when the potential power of the large machine was discovered, the manorial mill privilege was established. The home hand mills were banned. The Banal Rights gave the lords the sole power to operate mills; in early English law, for example, "mill soke" required that all subjects had to bring their grain to be milled in the village mill. Farmhouses were inspected, and illegal mills were destroyed.*

The big mill that was imposed on the people was eerie to them from the start. Often it was allowed to operate on Sundays or public holidays. The miller was allowed to work because the wind blows when and how it will, and the mill was dependent on the wind. Because the grain sacks accumulated during harvesttime, the miller had to grind day and night to keep up, regardless of the Christian calendar. The mill wheel rattled mercilessly, nonstop and without an organic rhythm. Often the gears ground loudly and creaked on after the normal work hours until late at night. Only on November 25, the day of Saint Catherine, the patron saint of millers, did the millwheel stand still, for on that day the saint had been martyred, dying on a breaking wheel, and it was believed that any miller who disregarded this law might die himself. It was preferable, therefore, to use this day to clean the millstones or tidy up the mill.

It is no wonder that the mill, which is out of sync with the god-given rhythm of days and nights, was considered a place where the devil was at work. Therefore, as a precaution, it was banished from the village and built on the outskirts of the settled area, or even farther away. In the Nordic languages, the mill is called *qvärn* or *kvern,* and folk etymology suggests it is an onomatopoeia that mimics the sound of wooden mechanics. In this word, matter groans as if tortured by spirits. The devil himself, it was said, comes to the mill at midnight. Dangerous spirits hung around there: at the watermills there were nixes or other water spirits; at the windmills, kobolds and similar entities.

---

*Similarly, other activities that once belonged to self-sufficient farmhouses or village communities, such as brewing and healing, were subject to the rule of the local lord, the church, or the state.

The mill outside the village was also considered a legitimate hostel for wayfarers and strays. The disreputable place, far from the prying eyes of the moral guardians, was also a place where people met for forbidden liasons or committed adultery. The beautiful miller's wife, according to the male fantasy of that time, kept busy with her guests and was well acquainted with "grinding"—a synonym for sexual intercourse. The Moulin Rouge, the Red Mill, is still the epitome of the sinful mill. The miller's wife appears not only as a seductress but often, in fairy tales and legends, as a witch who does her mischief in the form of a black cat. Her wanton activities can result in windstorms, floods, or mill fires.

Because the miller occasionally cheated the farmers over their flour, in many places he was suspected of being dishonest. After death, the door of heaven remains closed to him; he goes to hell or haunts as a ghost. But his dealings with the devil give him magical powers. He can, for example, staunch bleeding. A bleeding charm (from Westphalia) states:

> *Blut stehe still, still, still,*
> *Wie der ungerechte Müller es will.*
> *Im Namen des Vaters, des Sohnes . . .*

> Blood be staunched—stand still, still, still,
> As is the unfair miller's will.
> In the name of the Father, the Son . . .

Or another charm from Nuremberg (sixteenth century):

> *[Name], dir verstehe das Blut,*
> *als die Himmestür gegen einen ungerechten Müller tut.*

> [Name], may your blood close,
> like heaven's gate in front of a crooked miller's nose.

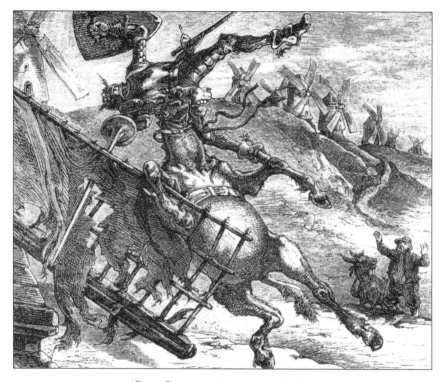

Don Quixote tilting at windmills

The mill, the high tech of its time, became a symbol of abandoning the divine order that is pleasing to God. The Spanish writer Miguel de Cervantes has the knight Don Quixote tilt at windmills in vain, and the 1931 movie version of *Frankenstein* lets the botched superman that was created by a power-hungry, insane scientist come to its end in a burning mill. In this case, the mill also stands for technology emancipated from the natural order of things.

Inquisition of Witches

In the early modern period, the European elite was literally obsessed with the idea of gears and powerful machines. Even God, the absolute being, was—as we have already seen—imagined as a rationally thinking machine builder. Even though man was physically only a machine, he had—thanks to his rational intellect—a share in the divine creative power. Constructing and operating machinery was therefore pleasing to God. It was considered modern to design everything optimally and efficiently according to rational mechanical principles: production processes for manufacturing, the market and economy, war campaigns, daily routines, ballroom dances, garden design, medicine, and the conduct of life in general.

By contrast, the miracles, superstitions, and spirits of the natural world—indeed, everything connected to traditional peasant culture— these backward beliefs were nothing but a hindrance that stood in the way of rational progress. It is no wonder that the witch hunt peaked in the sixteenth and seventeenth centuries. The burning of witches was above all a campaign, a crusade to eradicate magical (shamanic) thinking and perception (and it certainly did not hurt that the inquisitors were also allowed to confiscate their property). Among the rural folk, the wise women, shepherds, healers, midwives, and village magicians arrived at their knowledge in a way different from the new rationalists. Not only did these people safeguard older traditions and have excellent powers of observation, but they also received new insights through contemplation, rapture, or ecstatic communion with natural phenomena, slipping into these states and allowing themselves to be temporarily inspired by them. They explored the phenomena from the inside instead of measuring, calibrating, and analyzing it from the outside. In dreams and visions, the animals, the spirits of nature, and angels spoke to them.* Also, Mother Earth in the guise of Mary, for example, spoke to them and revealed her secrets. Of course, such a thing did not fit into the new worldview. The concept of superstition, which has roots in pre-Christian indigenous shamanism and is open to wide interpretation, was fought by church and state as a dangerous misconception. The nearly three hundred years of witch-hunting also gladly used the help of mechanisms. There were horrific machines in the torture chambers: vices, torture racks, thumbscrews, and breaking, or execution, wheels.

---

*What is referred to here should be clearly distinguished from the phenomenon of mentally unbalanced people who hear voices that are entirely the product of their own imagination.

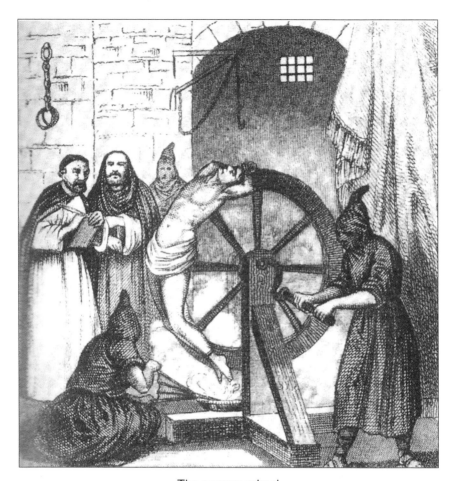

The torture wheel

Francis Bacon (1561–1626), the inventor of the controlled scientific experiment, founder of the inductive method, and *spiritus rector* of the Royal Society, was inspired by the witches' distressing interrogations.* For him, nature resembled a recalcitrant witch who had to be tormented with the help of mechanical devices such as levers, wheels, and screws into divulging its secrets. The researcher must lock nature

---

*The inductive method is based on the inference of a general conclusion (such as a law or theory) from a set of specific observations. By contrast, deduction starts with a general premise, which is then used to form specific conclusions.

into a laboratory and examine, analyze, and dissect it with the help of tools, because only then will they be able to control and improve it for the benefit of humanity (Merchant 1990, 179).

Can You Feel How Strong Your Heart Is?

Mills and clocks are the forerunners of later technologies that are increasingly changing our world. In 1712 the steam engine was invented, and in 1784 the first steam mill was built in London. The Industrial Revolution took its course. The British word for *factory* is "mill," as in a paper mill or steel mill, which in America is usually called a factory. In these mills human lives are also ground down. Society itself was structured like a machine; human life was rationally organized, and everyday existence became increasingly technologized—a process that not only continues today but also accelerates. Farms have even been transformed into countryside factories. Intensive pig fattening, dairy cattle concentration, and batteries of laying hens: meat, milk, and egg production accomplished according to a mechanical scheme. But we should realize that whatever is done to the animals will ultimately be done to humans, too. Why? Because the same underlying mind-set remains generally in force.

People have lost their faith in the natural course of things. As if the flowers do not grow on their own and the heart does not beat all by itself. Everything becomes optimized and controlled to the smallest detail, otherwise something might go wrong. There is a tendency to want to guard against anything that could go wrong, especially in human life.

Let's have a quick look at the typical life course of a human being in our technologized world. Birth in the hospital—a controlled technological process, without ecstasy, without mystery. Often the newborn baby is optimally cared for in the nursing station next to the mother, but if so it is separated from the mother, and thus from the rhythm of the maternal heartbeat, which accompanied it constantly in the abdomen. After struggling to see the light of the world, the little being needs the beating heart, the smell, the warmth of the mother. It should be carried in her arms, close to her body, and allowed to sleep by her side. The isolated baby's room, baby strollers, formula from a bottle instead of mother's milk, and pacifiers create a deep unconscious insecurity, a fear, and they cause a certain development of coldness in the heart from the very beginning. Nowadays one can place a heart sound machine—an electronic device that emits the calming sound of a heartbeat—in a baby's room or crib. The infant is supposed to believe there is a beating heart nearby. The soul of the baby surely recognizes the deception, however!

In most cases, the new mother must soon return to work in the office, in the shop, or in the factory. She is told that she is emancipated and that a job outside the home and away from the family will provide her with self-fulfillment. That may be true to some degree—or may not. Those who, like myself, grew up in the United States in the 1950s and 1960s can well remember what normal families were like. The man, the head of the family, was the breadwinner; he worked on his career until he had a heart attack or, at the very least, got ulcers.* Many women led a dreary life in the suburbs, feeling imprisoned and frustrated. There was not much to do in a fully automated household. Television entertainment and shopping often became the major occupation of their lives, and neurotic symptoms—a mania for cleaning and shopping, addiction to pills and alcoholism—were not uncommon. Grandma and Grandpa lived in senior apartments in sunny Florida or were otherwise cared for professionally in nursing homes. Traditional female labor that had existed from the Neolithic to the Industrial Revolution—such as cooking, caring for children, gardening, storing food for winter, caring for the sick in the family, brewing beer, laundry, sewing, spinning, weaving, gathering herbs, feeding animals, and whatever other chores needed to be done—was now increasingly performed by service providers or machines. Food and clothing were no longer produced by the women but instead bought

---

*Myocardial infarction and cardiovascular failure were at one time considered to be mainly associated with men's deaths, but since 1984 more women than men have been dying from these causes.

in stores. The children were in school full time. In a money economy, only money gives validity—and that was earned by the man of the household.

With the decline in purchasing power toward the end of the 1960s, it was soon necessary for both spouses to work so as to maintain their standard of living. "Home sweet home" began to vanish. In addition to snacks, TV dinners, and microwave meals, more than 50 percent of the daily meals are now consumed in fast-food restaurants. If the family can afford it, children are increasingly being looked after in day-care centers from a very young age. This is certainly a great relief for the parents; the little ones receive intellectual stimulation and can get some early practice in social interaction with peers and educational staff. One might ask, however, whether it allows for time to dream, to wonder and marvel, which is important for the development of a child's soul. And what about spontaneous and unregulated free time spent playing in nature, where plants, animals, and nature spirits are playmates and where one can directly experience one's surroundings without everything being mitigated through video, speech, and writing? The enormous performance pressure of attending all-day school often stretches children to their limits. The little free time that remains after schoolwork is then either provided with pedagogically meaningful activities—karate lessons, ballet class, baseball, riding lessons, afterschool programs—or the children retreat into the virtual world of their screens.

During puberty things can become quite precarious. A host of social workers and psychologists is needed to steer the rebellious young hearts into socially acceptable channels and guide their hormonal intoxication. The institutionalized pseudo-revolution of "sex, drugs, and rock'n'roll," sports, and recreation should help tone down and guide youthful demands. Underage drinking, drug use, and violence can be seen as the distress signals of troubled souls. Sooner or later, the rebels are usually brought back into the fold and reintegrated as taxpayers who fuel the mega machine—or as welfare recipients who depend upon it for survival. The sports and entertainment industries, whose stars earn millions, help to provide distractions and keep the pot boiling. A massive medical industry looks after the victims of the mega machine; the doctors serve as mechanics who keep the human work-machines functioning. After retirement, one can look forward to death. After the brain and nervous system shut down, all that is left is a slowly decomposing corpse that remains a disposal problem and a financial liability for the survivors. Today in modern, Western countries approximately 60 percent of the population dies in hospitals, and 30 percent die in nursing homes. The numbers are similar in other industrialized countries. The cause of death for nearly half of the people is cardiovascular failure.

This is, admittedly, a rather exaggerated characterization of the current life situation. But it nevertheless begs the question: Where can the human soul find meaning and orientation in such heartless times? Religious fundamentalism, hedonism, mindless consumption, or the flight into one utopia or another are some of the possibilities. The alternative subculture of the 1960s and 1970s attempted the latter. It has since been recognized that the gentle hippie dream of those times—Timothy Leary's "turn on, tune in, drop out" was completely unrealistic. Dropping out is virtually impossible. The machine is moving too fast.

Where is the answer? Poets and singers, like Marie Fredriksson (Roxette), call out: *Listen to your heart!* IC Falkenberg, a singer born in East Germany, sang in his 1989 ballad "Dein Herz" (Your Heart): *Fühlst du dein Herz—es schlägt für dich. / Fühlst du dein Herz—es kämpft um dich.* (Can you feel your heart—it is beating for you. / Can you feel your heart—it is fighting for you.)

Similarly, the wise tradition of India says that the wheel of *samsara,* the ever-changing karmic whirlwind within the space-time dimension in which we are trapped, can take on frightening dimensions. But in the middle of the storm, in the heart of being, in our own heart, there is calm and peace. There, the benevolent, peaceful, gracious divine Self (Christ, Shiva, Krishna, Buddha) lives. There we will find the peaceful source of love (*shanti*), and this love heals everything. So, we should go toward our heart, go into its divine center. That is the message.

THE HEART IS KING

In earlier times in our own culture, the mystery of the heart was also known. In the Renaissance, for example, there was the conception of the planetary gods: each of these deities had its own special task, in the great universe (macrocosm) as well as in the small one (microcosm); each was important, none could be left out. Each of the seven visible planets in the sky has its dwelling in a part of the cosmic primordial giant (macroanthropos), in the zodiac. This is also the case in the microcosm of the human body. Here, too, each planet has its habitation: the moon has its dwelling in the head, the sun in the heart, Jupiter in the liver, Mercury in the lungs, Venus in the kidneys, and so on. Each planet (each organ) has its task in the overall organism. Each one is important and plays its own part in the concert of life. However, the sun is the center—and that was the case even before Copernicus claimed that the earth and the other planets revolve around the sun. Already with the ancient Babylonians, the sun was described as the middle of the three superior and the three inferior planets. It was shown as the seat of a young king with a radiant crown. It gives light (enlightenment) and warmth (love) to the world. Wise Jupiter, ruler of the liver, is the old king who has withdrawn from active government and allows us to enjoy the pleasures of life. Mercury is the cunning, devious rogue next to the sun's throne and who dares to challenge the king's decisions with humor and wit. No matter how smart he is, he cannot put himself on the throne. Depending on one's perspective, the moon symbolizes dreamy or reflective consciousness, which is also an important component of wholeness. Lovely Venus plays a harmonizing role; Mars, the aggressive warrior, protects and defends; and ancient Saturn transforms life's experiences into crystalline wisdom.

Today we live in a time when we have forgotten the interplay of the inner planets. The head (intellect, cerebral function) has taken on the dominant role and subordinated and repressed the other planets. In our current cultural understanding, the mind is overvalued, and heart wisdom is undervalued.* But the heart is the one in the middle; it is the young king in us, it is light and soothing warmth. The planets must serve the sun; the head must serve the heart, and not the other way around.

Kopf ohne Herz macht böses Blut;
Herz ohne Kopf tut auch nicht gut.
Wo Glück und Segen soll gedeihn,
Muss Kopf und Herz beisammen sein.

Head without heart makes for bad blood;
Heart without head is also not good.
Where luck and blessings would abound,
Head and heart together should be found.

FRIEDRICH BODENSTEDT,
AUS DEM NACHLASSE DES MIRZA-SCHAFFY
(ENGLISH TRANSLATION
BY WOLF D. STORL)

---

*For the farmer-philosopher Arthur Hermes, my friend and mentor, it was clear that the overvaluation of the intellect is also the reason for the exaggerated sexualization and pornography of our modern culture. The hot, irrational sex instinct is the dialectical counterpart to the coolly calculating head. If the head is overvalued, the opposite pole must necessarily compensate. Unfortunately, the harmonizing, balancing middle—the heart— is missing in this kind of setup.

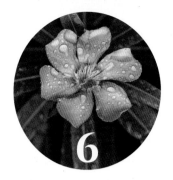

TRADITIONAL HEART PLANTS

Heart disease is not a mechanical defect, but an expression of our emotional state.

OLAF RIPPE, "DAS HERZ—
ORGAN DER SELBSTERKENNTNIS"
(THE HEART—ORGAN OF SELF-KNOWLEDGE)

THE TERM *TRADITIONAL HEART PLANTS* is used here to refer to those herbs, shrubs, and trees that were used to heal aggrieved hearts and heart ailments that accompanied states of sadness, melancholia, narrowheartedness, envy, hatred, lovelessness, or heartlessness. With these plants one usually searches in vain for cardiac glycosides, flavonoids, or alkaloids. From the modern point of view, then, one might say they have a psychogenic, or placebo effect. But placebos also heal, and they are often even amazingly effective. Maybe we should ask ourselves if we really understand what we so readily dismiss as a placebo. The ancestral, traditional heart plants appeal, above all, to the soul. They are part of the cultural morphogenetic field. Our ancestors, who are still somehow spiritually present in us, already knew these plants. Associated with the gods in pre-Christian times—and later with Mary, the Savior, and various saints—they point to sacred ground, to that which brings salvation; they can help to safeguard the soul and warm and calm the heart. The list of such traditional heart healing herbs is very long. Let us have a look at some of them here.

Bear Plants: Alpine Lovage (*Ligusticum mutellina*), Bear Leek (*Allium arsinum*), and Bearwort (*Meum athamanticum*)

The fear that modern humans have of bears is not only a sign of their alienation from nature itself but also from the nature of their own heart. Bears are—as those who know them will tell us—strong, fearless, and basically good-natured, and they know how to enjoy things. Humans should actually get along well with these shaggy companions. Encounters between humans and bears need not be a problem, provided that the human is calm and does not have a cowardly heart (Storl 2018a). My Cheyenne friend, Bill Tallbull, told me that, when the women and children went out into the wild in the fall to gather berries for drying in the winter, there were also bears around. They ate huge amounts of delicious wild fruit to help them get through their winter hibernation. The old medicine man told me that the bears were sometimes so close that the berry-pickers could hear them munching their food, and even smell them. They only become grouchy if they are disrespected by not allowing them the right-of-way. Bears can become seriously dangerous if they smell fear in a human being's scent; then they themselves become alert and are more likely to turn aggressive.

Most indigenous peoples admired the bear. It was considered a wild brother or an incarnate deity, a connoisseur of plants and a master of medicine. Its spirit gave strength to the shaman, healing powers to the healer, and courage to warriors. In the form of a beloved teddy bear, this creature still consoles and protects children when they are sad or lonely. Some historians of ancient history suspect that the cave bear, which was presumably mainly an herbivore, used to occasionally share winter quarters with humans and that its mere presence protected early humans from wolves, saber-toothed tigers, giant hyenas, and other predators (Storl 2018a, 23–24).

The natives of the European woodlands did not classify the plants according to planetary affiliation like the scholars of the Renaissance would later do, and certainly not according to the sexual characteristics of the flower organs, as scientists do today. They gave the plants totemic affiliations: wolf plants were corrosive and poisonous; horse plants were coarse and rough; dog plants were useless; the stork plants were children-bringers; and bear plants were big, usually hairy plants—the strongest of the medicinal plants, which bestowed fertility, gave people courage, and made the heart happy.

The bear plants belonged to the gods' bear, the *Asen*-bear, Ásbjörn (equivalent to the Anglo-Saxon name Osborn, "God-bear"), and this was none other than the strongest and most benevolent of the gods—namely, Thor (Old Norse Þórr; Anglo-Saxon Þunor). The bear-god brings on spring; as folklorists would say, the bear can also appear as a kind of grain spirit or vegetation numen.* With his lightning-striking paws and his rumble (spring thunderstorms), the bear-god drives away the winter torpor; the earth turns green and renews itself. The green spring herbs sprouting everywhere were always considered cleansing, rejuvenating, and renewing. The bear also eats them to regain his strength after his long winter hibernation. Thor drives out "worms"—that is, the demons of disease— he crushes them with his thunderbolt-hammer—he also annihilates "heart-worms" that feed on the vital life force.

We begin this chapter with some of the heart-strengthening bear plants: alpine lovage (*Ligusticum mutellina*), bear leek (*Allium arsinum*), and bearwort (*Meum athamanticum*).

---

*The grain spirits such as Korndämonen (grain demon), Feldgeister (field spirits), and other vegetation numina are among the mythical beings whose existence is not documented in older sources and which we only know from contemporary popular belief. The use of the word *demon* in this context does not necessarily refer to a malicious being that was demonized by the Christian Church but rather an entity or phenomenon that is considered supernatural in popular belief. Hence the more appropriate designation of "numen" as a personified supernatural or divine power.

Alpine Lovage
(*Ligusticum mutellina*)

Alpine lovage (*Ligusticum mutellina*), closely related to bearwort (page 150), grows in the Alps at altitudes of about 1,500 to 2,800 meters (4,921–9,186 ft.). Some of its Swiss and German common names include Madaun (from Latin *montana*), Alpen-Bärwurz (alp spignel), and Rahmbluem (cream flower, meaning if cows eat it their milk will be richer, creamier). Dairymen praise it as a grazing plant that helps the cows to produce plenty of good, creamy milk. Indeed, the alpine herders have a saying: "*Rispe, Muttern und Adelgras / sind die Beste, was die Kühli fraß*" (Panicle, alpine lovage, and alpine plantain are the best things our dear cows ate). In the folk medicine of the Alps, alpine lovage is considered one of the best stomach remedies and cardio-tonics.

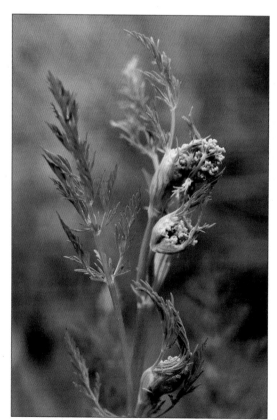

Alpine lovage (*Ligusticum mutellina*); the photo shows a young plant beginning to blossom in the spring.

The tea from the root is drunk three times a day to treat flatulence, dropsy, cough, stomach ailments, and heart failure. The plant has an antiviral effect. The Native Americans also knew a closely related plant from the *Lingusticum* genus, called osha, wild parsnip, or Porter's lovage (*Lingusticum porteri*). They called it bear medicine (*osha* = bear) in the Rocky Mountains. The aromatic root has the spirit of a bear, the Native Americans say, lending the warrior a strong, courageous heart.

Bear Leek
(*Allium ursinum*)

Bear leek (*Allium ursinum*), also known as bear's garlic, wild garlic, ramsons, buckram, or broad-leafed garlic, is a native of Europe and Asia. It grows in moist, deciduous forests and takes advantage of the time between snowmelt and the overall new foliage to shoot its sturdy green leaves as one of the first plants in the spring.*

Bear leek blooms at the end of April around the time of Walpurgis (April 30), at which time the leaves are no longer as juicy and tasty, and they die off toward the end of May. The underground bulbs remain dormant until the next spring. The seeds are distributed by ants. The plant's fresh green leaves and the pungent, sulfur-containing essential garlic oil that filled the air at that time of year were for the Celts, Germanic peoples, and Slavs a sure sign of the triumph of life over winter's deathlike grip. Such plants were so traditionally sacred for the Germanic peoples that they had a leek rune (ᛚ), the earliest name of which has been reconstructed as *laukaz*—the rune of living water and of the juicy, freshly budding vegetation. Appreciation of the plant is also evident from an example in Anglo-Saxon courtship: The young suitor recognized by the food that was served when he visited whether he would be accepted as a son-in-law. If beets were served, he could take his leave; if flour porridge was served, he was welcome as a friend; if the meal was pancakes

---

*A very similar species of wild leek in North America is *Allium tricoccum,* commonly known as ramps.

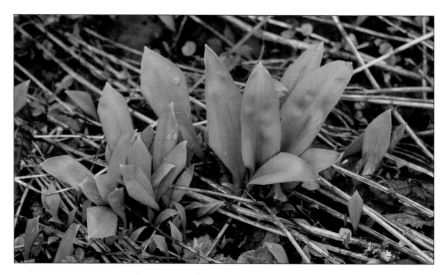

Bear leek (*Allium ursinum*) leaves

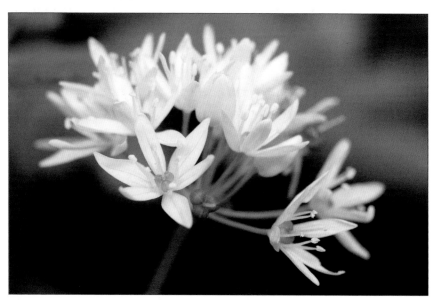

Bear leek (*Allium ursinum*) blossom

with bear leek, he had been accepted as a son-in-law. Among the Slavic peoples, bear leek, and later garlic from the Orient, was considered one of the best ways to ward off vampires. And even into modern times it is said that one should eat bear-leek soup on Walpurgis Night so that invisible roaming witches will leave one alone.

Bear leek can do everything that garlic (*Allium sativum*) does. The essential oils stimulate the secretion of gastric juice and bile, renew and regenerate the natural intestinal flora, and have an antispasmodic effect on stomach and intestinal cramps, as well as on the bronchi. Bear leek, like garlic, dilates the blood vessels and lowers blood pressure, which has a positive effect on arteriosclerosis. Both do so without the side effects (impotence, headache, etc.) of pharmaceutical blood pressure medication. Bear leek and garlic also improve lipid levels in the blood; they increase the proportion of good HDL cholesterol and reduce the oxidation tendency of LDL cholesterol. Garlic inhibits blood clotting by slowing the clotting tendency of platelets. In other words, bear leek and garlic protect against cardiovascular diseases.

Furthermore, the essential oil allicin strengthens the immune system; it promotes the propagation of natural killer cells, and it has a preventive effect against cancer, especially in the intestines (Weil 2000, 291). Allicin has an antibacterial and antifungal effect. It even works in a dilution of 1:10,000. For fungal diseases and for wound treatment, the juice can be applied externally. The essential oil is excreted mainly through the skin and the lungs (10 percent)—this can present a problem in social interaction—but as it passes through the lungs it cleanses, relaxes, and disinfects them. For this reason, garlic, or bear leek, simmered in milk, is also an excellent remedy for pneumonia.

For the Swiss herbalist pastor Johann Künzle (1857–1945) there was no other herb more effective than bear leek for cleansing the stomach,

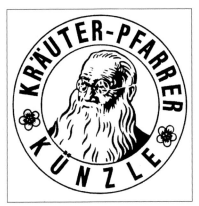

Swiss herbalist pastor
Johann Künzle

intestines, and blood. It provides the simplest and most pleasant spring blood-purification cure. "Chronically ailing people; people with eczema, boils, and rashes; the scrofulous and the anemic should value bear leek like gold. . . . With it, young people thrive and open like pinecones in the sun" (Künzle 1945, 358). He added: "The people of old gave it the name 'bear leek' because they saw that the bears, after their long hibernation, were weak and emaciated and ate massive amounts of this plant and soon regained their old strength" (Künzle 1911, 31).

Bearwort
(*Meum athamanticum*)

Bearwort (*Meum athamanticum*), also called baldmoney and spignel, is an umbellifer with extremely finely feathered aromatic leaves and a spicy root so hairy with brown fibers that it reminds one of a brown bear's fur. A native of central and western Europe, this little plant bear grows

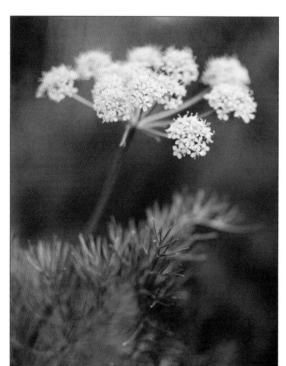

Bearwort (*Meum athamanticum*) leaves and blossom

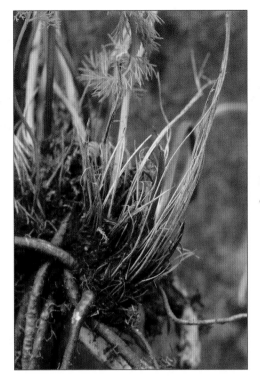

Bearwort (*Meum athamanticum*) roots

in rocky, lime-free soils above 23,000 feet. For Eurasian mountain farmers, it was practically a panacea. In the Black Forest in Germany, a bearwort schnapps (*Bärwurzschnaps*) is still distilled today. It is often kept in the traditional *Herrgottswinkel* (the Lord God's corner, a small altar in the northeast corner of the house) so that it is additionally charged with the power of the Blessed Mother and the saints. Bearwort schnapps is mainly used to treat uterine disorders; gastrointestinal complaints; and colds, coughs, and bronchial ailments. It is also used to strengthen a weak heart. Pierandrea Matthiolus, the Italian personal physician of Emperor Maximillian, mentioned it in 1563 as a cardiac-strengthening agent.

Blue Fragrant Violet
(*Viola odorata*)

Most violet species are native to the temperate regions of the Northern Hemisphere, though some are also found in widely divergent areas such

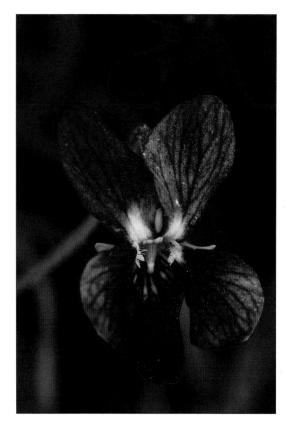

Blue fragrant violet
(*Viola odorata*)
blossom

as Hawaii, Australasia, and Peru. In Europe, there are about twenty-five species of violets. But because they pollinate each other and there are many bastardizations, no botanist can really tell how many types of violets actually exist. Apart from yellow and white violets, folk medicine refers to only two: blue fragrant violets in the spring and dog violets (or heath dog violets), which bloom spring to early summer. The fragrant violet is suitable for healing, but the dog violet is not ascribed with any healing power.

The beautiful blue-purple flower color and the beguiling scent have always attracted attention. The violet is a herald of spring, that longed-for time in the northern world, when the cold and dead of winter ceases for humans and beasts, and the heart can rejoice. We know it from a German song composed by Amadeus Mozart and Christian Overbeck, which became so popular that it is now considered a traditional folk song:

Komm lieber Mai und mache die Bäume wieder grün,
und lass mir an dem Bache ein Veilchen wieder blühen!
Wie möchte ich doch so gerne ein Blümchen wieder
sehen.
Ach, lieber Mai wie gerne einmal spazieren gehen.

Come on, dear May, and let the trees turn green once
more,
and let the violets bloom for me by the brook!
How I would like to see a flower again.
O, dear May, how gladly would I go out again for a
stroll.

In many rural areas of Europe, it was the custom that whoever found the first violet in the spring ran through the village and proclaimed the good news. Violet leaves were part of the spring meal—the soup made of fresh, green wild plants that was cooked to purify and renew the blood, which was a spring tradition already in pre-Christian times. By eating the soup, spring was also invited right into the body. The purple flowers, which smell sweet but taste sour, were also eagerly collected. In the Middle Ages they were used as medicine and for seasoning and coloring vinegar. In later times, especially in the eighteenth and nineteenth centuries, they were used in the production of jelly, marmalade, and pastilles (scented kisses); the flowers were candied, put into liqueur, syrup, ice cream, and eau de toilette. Fortunately, collecting the small plant does no harm. Not only is it a perennial that reproduces through root sprouts, but the fragrant March flowers are also usually sterile and do not produce seeds. Much later in the year, they flower once again, but these are dwarf blossoms, which hide under the leaves and do not even open completely. They pollinate themselves and then produce many seeds. The seeds are provided with fatty and protein-rich appendages (elaiosomes) so that they attract ants, which then spread them.

The beautiful flowers were categorized in the humoral medicine of

Hippocrates and Galen as cool and moist. Their effect was said to be soothing, to help make acrid fluids milder, to stimulate discharge, to calm, and to act as a slight laxative. Violets were believed to strengthen the heart; to ward off malignancy and black bile (melancholia); and to heal epilepsy, mental confusion, fever, coughing, headaches, and ulcers (Ingo Müller 1993, 220). The ancient Greeks knew a violet heart-drink to treat heated outbursts of anger and insomnia and to calm the heart. A violet head wreath is also said to relieve a hangover and to cool the head.

One of the grandfathers of German herbalism, Hieronymus Bock (sixteenth century), prescribed it for all "hot" diseases, such as stitches, headaches, and liver inflammation. He wrote: "Viola . . . keeps the belly open [working well] and strengthens the heart" (Bock 1539). Hildegard of Bingen recommended the violet for melancholy, dull eyes, and cancer. Otto Brunfels used violet petals and violet water for fever, tumors, and a "heated" liver. In addition, it was claimed to stop stomachache and heart pains and to drive fiery anger out of the brain. The English herbalist Nicholas Culpeper confirmed that "a dram weight of the dried leaves or flowers of Violets, but the leaves more strongly, doth purge the body of choleric humours" and "the dried flowers of Violet are accounted among the cordial [relating to the heart] drinks." The remedy "eases pain in the head, caused through want of sleep, helps quinsy (tonsillitis) and epilepsy, and refreshes the sense of life" (Culpeper 1999, 188). Culpeper, convinced of the planets' influence on the plants, placed the violet under the rule of mild Venus. Rudolf Steiner saw, above all, the effect of Mercury in violets. "The violet is 'all nose.' It absorbs the odor of Mercury. We smell Mercury in violets" (Pelikan 1975, III:241).

In the past, a strong decoction of violet roots was considered an excellent emetic that helped to purge a disease. South American ipecacuanha (*Cephaelis ipecacuanha*), which also has a strong irritant effect on the stomach lining, later replaced the violet root as an emetic in Western countries. Folk medicine still recognizes violet tea as a gargle for inflamed tonsils and laryngeal ulcers. Also, the saponin-containing tea or syrup is still used as an expectorant.

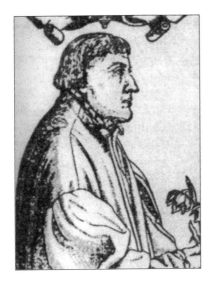

German grandfather of
botany and herbalism,
Hieronymus Bock
(1498–1554)

Many legends surround this delicate and fragrant flower. Wherever it grew, it was cherished. The northern Germanic peoples consecrated it to the god Tyr. For Mohammed, it embodied the glory of Islam; it is the Prophet of the Rose just as the rose is the Prophet of Allah. For the ancient Greeks, the violet was seen as having been the lovely daughter of the Titan Atlas; when Apollo demanded her, she withdrew from his approach by transforming herself into this flower. Elsewhere, it was said that the violet originated after Zeus, the father of the gods, had turned his young lover Io into a cow to protect her from the jealousy of his wife, Hera. (Unfortunately, that did not help because Hera then plagued the cow in the form of a gadfly.) So that the beloved cow would also have something worthy to eat, Zeus let a pasture of fragrant violets sprout.

Despite the fact that, in antiquity, the love goddess Aphrodite was called the violet-haired and at her wild festivals people adorned themselves with violet wreaths, the violet was considered a flower of innocence and of virgins. The motif was adopted and taken further by the Christians: God had created this flower to provide the pious with a picture of humility. For the Christians, the violet even became a symbol of the Crucified One himself. It recalls of the patiently endured humiliation of the Savior, and the flower's purplish-blue color suggests the purple robe that his tormentors put on him during the Passion. In Vienna in the twelfth century it was recorded that the violets, which were gathered in spring for the ruling house from meadows by the Danube, were only allowed to be picked by innocent virgins.

The violet, which blooms so close to the undergrowth, also belonged to the death goddess Persephone, who dominated the subterranean kingdom with her dark master, Pluto. That is probably why coffins and graves were adorned with violets in antiquity. The Slavic Wends told of how the daughter of their rich, treasure-laden underworld god Chernobog grew, unrecognized, as a violet. Every ten years on Walpurgis Night, for a brief time she takes on her true form as an enchantingly beautiful maiden. Whoever finds and plucks the flower in the night, before she transforms herself, wins her as a wife and has access to the hidden treasures of Chernobog.

Bog Star
(*Parnassia palustris*)

The bog star, commonly known as grass-of-parnassus, is not noticed much nowadays.* It is closely related to the Saxifragaceae family and grows in arctic and alpine conditions, as well as in wet meadows, bogs, and marshes across the entire Northern Hemisphere. The delicate flower is named after its star-like blossoms, whereas its German common name *Herzblatt* (heart leaf) refers to the shape of its leaves. It is likely due to this signature of the leaves that the herb was once used as a tea for nervous heart palpitations. The Cheyenne make an infusion from the powdered dry leaves of the very similar *Parnassia fimbriata* (fringed grass of Parnassus), which they use to treat gastrointestinal problems.

---

*This herb from the Parnassiaceae family, which occurs in the Northern Hemisphere, should not be confused with the heart leaf (*Mentzelia cordifolia*) native to Peru. The Indians use the latter plant as an effective stomach remedy, and it is now sold in German pharmacies as Anguraté stomach tea.

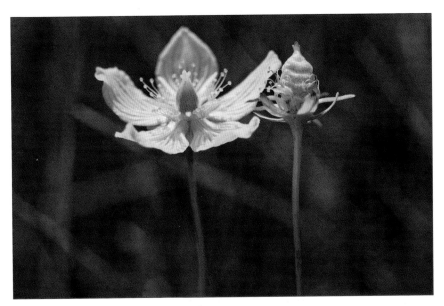

Bog star (*Parnassia palustris*) blossom and fruit

Borage
(*Borago officinalis*)

The mere sight of flowering borage in the garden, with its beautiful, sky-blue, star-shaped flowers, is good for heart and soul. The devout Christians in northern Europe dedicated this plant—which is native to the Mediterranean and was later planted in cloister gardens in the north—to the Blessed Virgin Mary, who, as the mistress of nature, wore a blue cloak decorated with stars.*

The blue flowers are the color of the seventh heaven, the firmament, the sphere where Saturn—the outermost planet that is visible to the naked eye—has its orbit. This saturnine blue, which we also find in the flower of the closely related forget-me-not (*Myosotis palustris*), evokes feelings of the distant horizon, of homesickness or wanderlust, of yearning, and sometimes of sadness and melancholy. It is the wild

---

*A sky-blue cloak was also worn by Freya, the ancient Germanic goddess, and likewise by the shamanic female seeresses of early Germanic societies, such as the Norse *völvur* (sg. *völva*), or the continental Germanic seeress named Veleda.

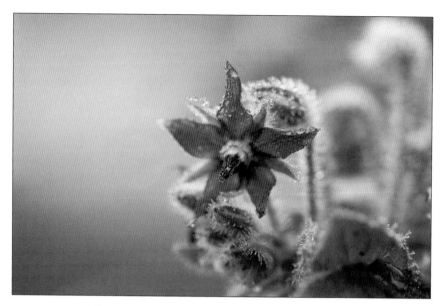

Borage (*Borago officinalis*) leaves and blossoms

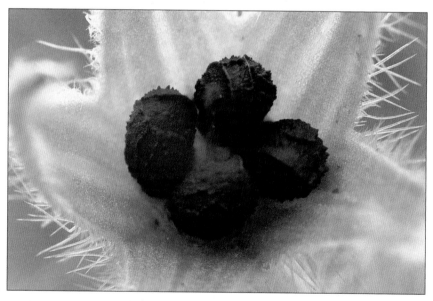

Borage (*Borago officinalis*) seeds

blue yonder, the things that come out of the blue, the elusive blue flower of romance, and the feeling of having the blues. Blue-flowering borage was considered a homeopathic remedy for such melancholic, wistful moods. Therefore, it was also called *Euphrosinon* in antiquity, which the learned clergymen translated as "gladness." Hieronymus Bock, one of the fathers of botany, wrote that the borage plant should be eaten by "dull-witted and weak persons," and he suggests "to drink the lovely flowers as tea, so that weak, sad people may forget their sufferings" (Bock 1539, 157).

The Romans said about this plant, *ego borago, gaudi semper ago* (I, borage, always further a good mood), and liked to steep the flowers in their wine. Courage and joie de vivre are the main characteristics of a strong heart. Again and again, one reads in the old herbals that borage strengthens the heart. For example, Tabernaemontanus states: "The flowers, eaten raw and in a drink, thereafter, calm a nervous heart" or "the lovely borage flowers should be used liberally in food and drink.... They strengthen the heart and brain; awaken despondent, mournful, melancholy people to joy and lightheartedness; and purify the blood" (Tabernaemontanus 1588–1591).

For the humoral doctors of the Middle Ages who defined diseases as an imbalance of the four humors—yellow bile (*cholera*), black bile (*melancholera*), blood (*sanguis*), and phlegm (*phlegma*)—borage was classified as warm and moist. The plant is purifying, softening, balances melancholic humors, and mitigates yellow bile. In other words, it dispels sadness (melancholia) and anger (the choleric emotion) from the heart. In addition, it strengthens the memory as well as the heart, drives out poisons from the *spiritus,* and cheers the mood (Ingo Müller 1993, 152). The pharmacists of antiquity included borage—together with violet, woodruff, and rose—as one the four heart-strengthening blossoms, the *Quatuor flores cordiales.* This is why, in Germany, the common folk gave the plant—which now had spread and grew outside the cloister gardens—names like *Herzblümlein* (little heart flower), *Herzfreude* (heart's joy), or *Herzblume* (heart blossom). Because the edible young, rough, hairy leaf tastes a bit like cucumber, the Dutch also call it cucumber flower (*konkommerbloem*). In Styria (Austria), the herb is called *Beinlfutter* (honeybee food) because of its nectar-rich flowers, and in St. Gallen (Switzerland) it is called *Jumpfergsichtli* (maiden's face).

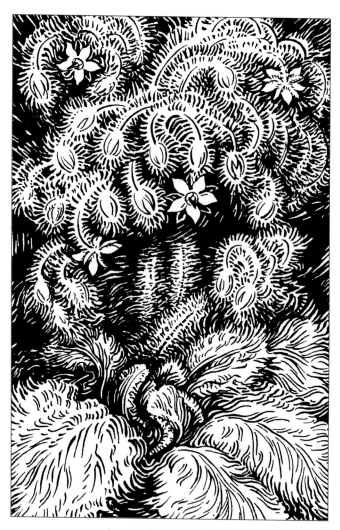

Borage (*Borago offinalis*)

Linguists can't agree about the origin of the word *borage*. Some say the word comes from the Arabic *abu 'araq*, "father of sweat," as it was used in the Middle East as a blood-cleansing sudorific to expel bad body fluids. It is more likely that the name comes from Italian *borra* ("hairy, bristly," from Latin *burra*, "shaggy garment"). That would be very appropriate for this bristly member of the borage family (Boraginaceae). Other etymologists seek the origin in the Celtic-Gaelic word *borrach*, which means "proud man." And finally, some suppose that we are dealing with a corruption of *corago* (*cor, cordis,* "heart" + *ago,* "to act on"), "acts on the heart" (thus similar to another of the plant's common names in Germany: *Herzstärker,* "heart strengthener").

We know that borage slightly lowers blood pressure because it helps the blood vessels relax, but it has no direct influence on the pumping mechanism. There are also no psychotropic alkaloids that act on brain or nerve functions. Borage is, above all, a stress-reducing agent. It supports the function of the adrenal cortex, the endocrine gland that provides about fifty hormones of various kinds to the body. These include sex hormones and hormones involved in stress responses; steroid hormones used in the regeneration of cells; and cortisones, which have an anti-inflammatory and anti-allergic effect. Borage has an anti-melancholic effect when life in general is just getting one down. By supporting the renal glands, it has a regulating and regenerating effect on convalescents after cortisone and steroid treatments. Because it influences the sex hormones, it makes sense that in folk medicine women would mix borage leaves into tossed salads when they wanted to become pregnant. The leaves and seeds also stimulate the milk flow for nursing mothers. The herb, taken as a tea, is otherwise a mild sudorific and blood-purifying agent for the elimination of wastes in the body. Furthermore, borage—which contains tannins; silicic acid; mucilage; and diuretic, antiseptic-acting asparagine—was traditionally administered as an infusion to treat colds, coughing, sore throat, and pneumonia. Externally, the crushed fresh herb can be applied to ulcers, eczema, hives, insect bites, and abscesses.

The thick black seeds of the annual plant are dispersed by myrmecochory (from ancient Greek *mýrmēx,* "ant" + *choreiā,* "circling motion"), which means—as is the case with violets, for example—that ants diligently spread them around. It has recently been discovered that oil made of the seeds is somewhat of a superfood. It contains as much as 25 percent gamma-linolenic acid (GLS), an unsaturated, essential fatty acid that, among other things, helps the body to produce prostaglandin. Studies show that this gamma-linolenic acid—which is incidentally also found in the seeds of black currants, hemp, and evening primrose—is helpful for treating polyarthritis, endogenous eczema, premenstrual syndrome (PMS), hay fever, brittle hair and nails, dry skin, lacrimal gland ailments (Sjögren's syndrome), and even multiple sclerosis (Phaneuf 2005, 57; Mabey 1993, 89).

A flower essence, inspired by the essences of Edward Bach, has also been produced from borage blossoms. It is said to strengthen the heart and increase optimism (McIntyre 2919, 75). In the flower language of the Middle Ages, wearing or giving a blossoming borage stem meant loyalty, sincerity, and good courage. In her *Liederbuch* (Songbook), written down in 1471, the scribe Clara Hätzerlin from Augsburg, Germany, includes the following:

> Whoever's heart is free of all malice and stands up for full justice should wear borage. The herb is rough and does not break easily, but all the freer stands the blossom and quickens sick hearts. (Zacharias 1982, 31)

An aphorism of Mr. Stanislao Reinhardo Axtelmeier (Augsburg, 1705) reads: "This herb is quite the heart-herb; it creates joy and good courage and drives away sadness" (Zacharias 1982, 31). One cannot help but think that borage might be just the right herb for the times we are living in today!

Chamomile
(*Matricaria chamomilla*)

Chamomile is a plant of the sun. Like the daisy, it delights the heart and the senses. With its little domed yellow flower head, ringed by a bright garland of radiant white flower petals, it is reminiscent of a small sun shining in the light-blue sky. The finely feathered leaves are perfectly light permeated: they have cast off any heavy, watery, moonlike mass and suggest a predisposition to the order-giving cosmic forces of light. The flowers are very sun loving—at night and in cloudy weather or rain, they close and hang their heads. In the bright days of summer, they bloom the most and smell the strongest. Not surprisingly, they

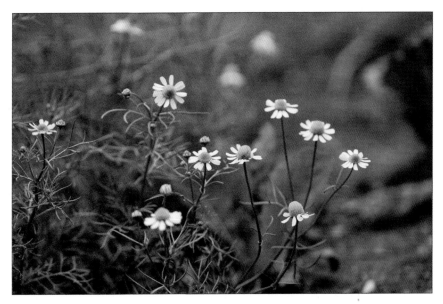

Chamomile (*Matricaria chamomilla*) blossoms

were dedicated to the sun god Baldur, whose "eyelashes are as gentle and graceful as the ornamental petals of the chamomile" (Zerling 2007, 133). It is one of the nine herbs of Woden (Wotan, Odin), with which this shamanic god of healing conquered the decay- and disease-causing serpent (Storl 2005a, 282).

Chamomile has always been a mothers' plant (as its Latin name *Matracaria* indicates), a female herb, and has been known as a healing herb since the Stone Age. Even today, it is the most popular general herbal remedy in central Europe. It is above all the streaming midsummer light that finds expression in the splendid healing power of chamomile. Its effects reach into the depths of the body, including the mucous membranes of the intestines, lungs, and female reproductive organs. Everywhere where mucus and pus are produced, where dissipative factors that irritate the tissues are at work, it sets its ordering, cosmic light effect into motion to heal these things. It soothes, cleanses, calms, disinfects, relieves spasms and pain, and promotes healing. It works into the soul and touches the heart—albeit on the etheric-energetic level, rather than one that results from an active constituent.

The effects of chamomile are also scientifically proven today: it calms, as it contains flavonoids that bind to GABA receptors (similar to benzodiazepine tranquilizers). It contains substances (for example, tetracoumaroyl spermine) that block pain receptors. And the bisabolol contained in the plant is anti-inflammatory, antispasmodic, anxiolytic (fear-reducing) and calming (Phaneuf 2005, 71).

Daisy
(*Bellis perennis*)

The daisy is native to western, central, and northern Europe but has become naturalized in most temperate regions, including the Americas and Australasia. It contains saponins, tannins, flavonoids, mucilaginous substances, some essential oil, and organic acids, which together have a detoxifying, metabolizing, expectorant, and mildly anticonvulsant effect. That is why, in phytotherapy, we find an infusion of the flowers used as a cough suppressant and to treat skin diseases, gastrointestinal complaints, and liver disease. As a heart remedy, however,

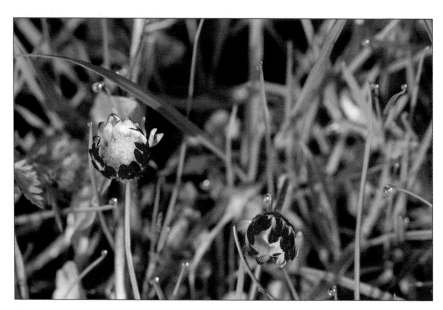

Daisy (*Bellis perennis*) blossoms

it is unknown today. Yet the pretty, unassuming blossom touches our hearts. In German the plant is called goose flower (*Gänseblümchen*) because it grew on the village green, where the young women used to herd the geese. It was once dedicated to the goddess Freya, who, like a goose maiden, herds and watches over human souls.

The daisy was also called the eye of the sun, Baldur's eyebrow, or simply day's eye (Old English *dæges ēage*, whence came the modern English "daisy") because the flowers are completely connected with the sun's rhythm, with the heart of the macrocosm: the flowers turn with the sun and open only in the sunshine. The sight of the daisy dispels all sadness and darkness from the soul. The English poet Chaucer (ca. 1342–1400) praised it and wrote that every morning in May he gets up early in the morning and looks at the blooming daisies in the meadow, because only they "could ease his sadness."

It is said that if one can step on seven daisies with the sole of one foot, then spring is finally here and the cold, nasty winter season is truly over. The first three daisies, which are found in the spring, are considered particularly curative; they protect from fever, the evil eye, and toothache all year long—but they must be bitten off and not touched with the hand. The roots of the flower, worn as an amulet, lend affection, happiness, and understanding.

The daisy is a children's plant. Girls used to wear daisy wreaths in their hair and wove the flowers into necklaces. Daisies symbolize innocence, gentleness, and a pure heart.

Hedge Woundwort
(*Stachys sylvatica*)

Whoever has sniffed it once will not forget the hedge woundwort, also known as hedge nettle or whitespot. The strong scent of the heart-shaped leaves of this member of the Lamiaceae family, native to Europe and Central Asia, can be described as earthy, spicy, unpleasant, and fetid. In folk medicine, the forest plant was used externally to treat gland tumors and internally to relieve diarrhea, colic, and menstrual cramps. The herb

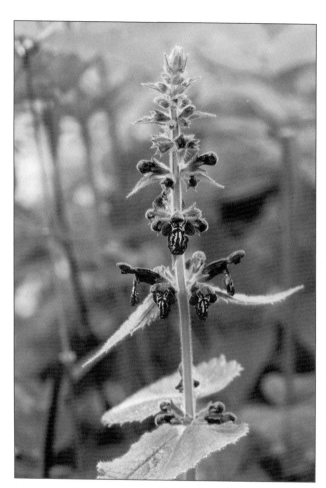

Hedge woundwort
(*Stachys sylvatica*)
leaves and
blossoms

was boiled into a broth, or crushed leaves were mixed with vinegar and applied to heal festering wounds. In Germany it was considered one of the heathen woundworts (*heidnische Wundkräuter*), which meant that its efficacy was so marked that even our pagan ancestors were aware and made use of it. The essential oil that it exudes has an antibacterial effect. The hedge woundwort is also what in German is called an enchantment herb (*Berufkraut*)—meaning that if children or animals have been bewitched or enchanted, they can be bathed in a decoction of the plant and thus freed of the spell. There are many plants in this category, and hedge woundwort is one of them. Farmers would bathe the cows' udders with hedge woundwort tea if they were not giving as much milk as they should, or if the udder was infected or ailing. The herb was burned as incense or buried under the doorsill to drive away evil spirits. It is also said to help with cramps in the feet caused by evil spirits.

Hardly anyone today knows this forest plant, although it is still quite widespread. Its uses have likewise been forgotten. It is interesting to note that in earlier times a distilled water of the flowers was used "to make the heart merry, to make a good colour in the face, and to make the vitall spirits more fresh and lively" (Grieve 1981, 862). In his large book on herbal remedies, the herbalist pastor Johann Künzle wrote: "The hedge woundwort possesses as many heart-strengthening powers as the poisonous foxglove without having its side effects" (Künzle 1945, 484). However, no one seems to have followed this advice so far.

Key Flower
(*Primula veris, P. officinalis*)

For the ancient Germanic peoples, the tuft of sun-yellow key flower resembled a bunch of keys, just as the housewife, the mistress of the farmstead, used to wear on her belt, which gave her access to all the chambers and chests. It is a native of temperate Europe and western Asia and a member of the primrose family, commonly called primrose or cowslip. In this wildflower—whose medieval German name is attested as *himelslüzzel* (heaven's key)—the northern peoples of Europe would have recognized the ring of keys belonging to Freya, the beautiful goddess of life, love, and pleasure. The name Freya, like the German word *Frau,* means "the lady." She alone has the power to lock and unlock the cosmic periods of time. Every year, with her golden flower keys, she opens the locked-up heavenly chamber and frees the springtime—the warm, blissful season. With these keys she also opens people's hearts, so that the joy of life can enter once more after the long, cold winter.

The Christian missionaries took this ring of keys from the heathen goddess and gave it to Saint Peter, the master of the weather and guardian of the pearly gates. He opens the pearly gates for the devout and sends the sinners away. One day, according to a popular folktale,

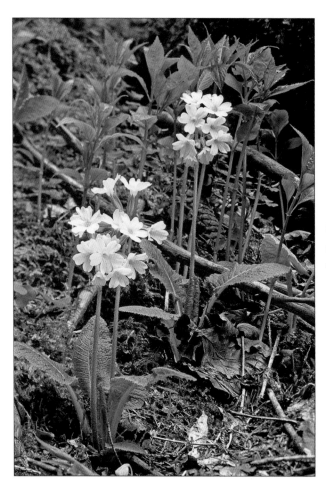

Key flower or cowslip (*Primula veris*) in full bloom

the devil tried to sneak into heaven. Stealthily, he crept up to the gates. When Saint Peter saw the devil's shadow, he was so frightened that his key ring slipped from his hand and fell to the ground, and when the keys touched the ground, they turned into key flowers. *Herba Sancti Petri* or *Petrusschlüssel* (St. Peter's keys) are two medieval names for key flower. Because the plant was believed to have fallen from heaven, it was considered helpful in treating epilepsy and dizziness. Tightrope-walkers wore the flower as an amulet so that they could keep their balance at lofty heights without fear of falling. Important herbalists of the sixteenth century, such as Pietro Mattioli or Hieronymus Bock, prescribed distilled cowslip water to treat cases of dizziness and strokes.

Hildegard of Bingen recommends the beautiful cowslip primrose as a heart medicine:

> Primrose (*hymelslozel*) is hot. . . . [It] takes its strength especially from the power of the sun, whence it checks melancholy. When melancholy rises in a person, it makes him sad and agitated in his moods. It makes him pour forth words against God. Airy spirits notice this, and rush to him, and by their persuasion turn him toward insanity. This person should place primrose on his flesh, near his heart, until it warms him up. The airy spirits dread the primrose's sun-given power and will cease the torment. (Hildegard of Bingen 1998, 91–92)

In modern phytotherapy, the roots and blossoms of the key flower are used mainly to treat colds and chronic bronchitis. The plant has even received a positive monograph from Commission E.*

Lemon Balm
(*Melissa officinalis*)

Many people are familiar with lemon balm. The perennial, heat-loving plant, a member of the Lamiaceae family, which flowers from midsummer to August, grows in many gardens. The plant is a native to south-central Europe, the Mediterranean Basin, Iran, and Central Asia, but nowadays it is known worldwide. On warm days, the whole plant smells wonderfully of lemon, which has earned it the name lemon balm. The plant absorbs a large amount of light and heat and then passes them on to us in the form of an essential oil. North of the Alps, it is not a native. Monks brought plants from the Meditarranean region and nursed them

---

*Commission E was a panel of experts established in 1978 by the Federal Health Office of (West) Germany. Their task was to determine pharmaceutical quality, effects, side effects, interactions, and indications of medicinal plants according to scientific criteria. The plants examined received either a positive or a negative profile (monograph). The commission continued operating in Germany until 1995 (Bühring 2007, 10).

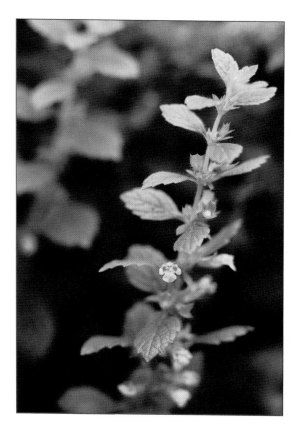

Lemon balm
(*Melissa officinalis*)
leaves and blossoms

Saturn, bringer of
misfortune (illustration
from a German
calendar, Basel, 1514)

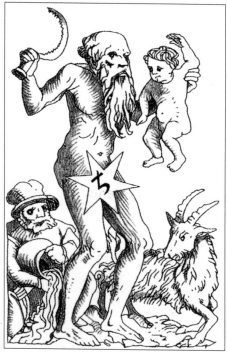

in their monastery gardens. For this reason, there are hardly any Celtic or Germanic traditions, legends, or popular beliefs regarding this aromatic herb. However, people soon became convinced of the healing power of this *Pfaffenkraut* ("priest's herb," a derogatory German folk name for the plant) and Charlemagne (747–814), Holy Roman Emperor (800–814) and conqueror of the pagan continental Saxons, ordered the cultivation of lemon balm on all lands in his empire.

Hildegard of Bingen was enthusiastic about the *Binsuga-Apiago* (Middle High German for "bee suckle"; Latin *apis,* "bee"), as she called lemon balm. She claimed it has the power of fifteen other herbs in it. She writes: "Whoever eats it will readily laugh because its warmth subdues the spleen and the heart becomes joyful" (Marzell 2002, 205). The then prevalent humoral theory of medicine labeled as "heart diseases" things such as gloominess, sadness, nightmares, and the inability to laugh heartily; they were believed to be an effect of melancholy vapors rising from the spleen and clouding the heart and brain. The ruler of the spleen is the leaden, gloomy, morose Saturn. The fragrant sweet lemon balm, however, is under the rule of Jupiter—the doctors of antiquity had no doubt about that. Like the sun, Jupiter is also a protector against Saturn's negative influences.

Like other herbalists, Hildegard saw the signature of the heart in the leaf shape. The grandfathers of German botany and herbalism—Brunschwig (1500), Brunfels (1532), and Bock (1539)—also called lemon balm a heart wort. Paracelsus called it a heart comforter (*Herztrost*). He writes: "Of all things the earth produces, lemon balm is the best herb for the heart" (Sudhoff 1922–1933, IX:322). Pietro Andrea Mattioli, court physician of Emperor Maximilian II, informs us: "Lemon balm has a wonderfully good way of strengthening and refreshing the heart, especially when it is frightened, beating fast at night and disturbing peaceful sleep. It purifies the blood; reverses displeasure and melancholic sadness; does service to the cold, damp stomach and nearly all internal organs" (Mattioli 1563, 347d).

The humoral theory described lemon balm as warm and dry to the second degree (regarding the degrees of the humoral system, see the

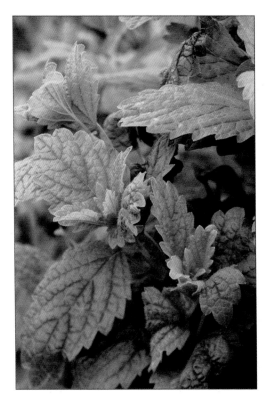

Lemon balm
(*Melissa officinalis*)
fresh shoots

footnote on page 23) and fortifying for the heart, brain, and uterus. Thus, it is also a flower for female disorders. In German one of its common names is *Mutterwurz* (motherwort). In earlier times, the term *mother* also meant the uterus. Brunfels, in his *Contrafayt Kreüterbuch* (1532, 302), also called the plant a motherwort and woman's herb (*Frauenkraut*) because "it was much used by women for the uterus" (*es zu der mutter bei den frawen hefftig gebraucht würt*). In the early German herbal *Gart der Gesundheit* it says that *Melissa* (lemon balm) "cleanses the uterus and gives women the strength to give birth" (Schöffer 1485).

Other herbals state as well that lemon balm, as a woman's herb and in the right dosage, regulates menstruation, promotes conception, dampens states of sexual overstimulation, relieves premenstrual syndrome, and has a calming effect for menopause. Both lemon-balm tea and *Melissengeist* (an alcoholic extract of lemon balm) are supposed to help relieve inner agitation when one is secretly in love, confusion of the heart, butterflies in the stomach, lovesickness, and, of course, hysteria. Hysteria (from Greek *hustéra,* "uterus"), a medical term from the eighteenth century, describes the condition in which the sexually unsatisfied uterus supposedly somehow travels up through the body to the head and thereby produces confused thoughts, heart palpitations, and migraines.

In antiquity, lemon balm was dedicated to the goddess Demeter and her daughter Persephone. Incidentally, the priestesses of Demeter were called *Melissae,* meaning "honeybees." Beekeepers still treasure *Melissa officinalis* as a friend to this day. In German lemon balm is called *Zitronen Melisse* (lemon melissa), and other German names, such as *Bienenfang* (bee catcher) and *Immekraut* (beekeeper's herb), clearly show the connection. This mint species is not just a good honey plant for bees; it also contains a pheromone that attracts them. For that reason, beehives—which were already in use by the ancient Romans—are rubbed down with lemon balm, or some plants are placed on the hive.

But the plant was dedicated not only to Demeter. Lemon balm was primarily the cult plant of the wild virgin goddess Artemis, the mistress of the female source of life, especially in her later identification with Eileithyia, the goddess of childbirth. The Greek physician Dioscorides (ca. 40–90 CE), who wrote the Western world's first herbal, already cited lemon balm as a gynecological remedy—for example, as a decoction in a sitz bath for the purification of the mother (uterus) (Marzell 1943–1979, III:131). The Christians adopted this sacred plant of the ancient goddesses and made it the attribute of Mary, the perpetual virgin "from whom comes all sweetness."

The Christian Church has always been a friend of "spirits"—after all, the blood of the Incarnate God was identified with fermented grape juice—that is, red wine. Therefore, it is not surprising that monks and priests, who, since the High Middle Ages, also had access to Arabic alchemical writings, were very active in distilling herbal spirits and liqueurs. After the Reformation, many former monks who had lost their positions in the church and were consequently unemployed began to distill and sell alcoholic elixirs. Lemon balm played a major role in this practice. It was within this tradition that Discalced Carmelites secretly distilled the herbal tonic in Paris in 1611 that later became known as Carmelite Water or *Melissengeist* and which remains popular in Germany to this day. In addition to lemon balm, the clear brew contains lemon peel, nutmeg, angelica root, betony, coriander, cloves, and cinnamon. In 1826, Maria Clementine Martin, who had been put into the care of the Carmelite nunnery in Cologne by her father, established the Klosterfrau brand of *Melissengeist,* which has since become a comfort to many women. This lemon balm liqueur consoled her and her sisters with respect to the cheerless monastic life whose rules demanded poverty, humility, chastity, and fasting. Today, *Melissengeist* is rarely produced from the lemon balm plant itself. The pure essential oil is far too expensive—one liter costs more than $20,000! The precious lemon balm essence is usually replaced by the essential oil (lemon oil) of East Indian lemongrass (*Cymbopogon winterianus*).

Modern research confirms the soothing effect of lemon balm as a phyto tranquilizer for nervous ailments, migraines, nervous heart complaints, stomach cramps, and intestinal disorders. The essential oils (citral, geranial, neral) have an antispasmodic effect via the limbic system. In addition, there is a proven virus-inhibiting effect due to phenolic acids and polyphenols, which is why it is good as a tea for colds or mumps and as an ointment-ingredient for herpes, shingles, blisters, and cold sores. Lemon balm leaves in a sachet, or as an additive to a bath, soothe and relax as well. However, because lemon balm slightly inhibits thyroid function, someone who suffers from hyperthyroidism should use it with caution. The latest neuropharmacological research suggests that lemon balm could also help with Alzheimer's disease (Phaneuf 2005, 217).

Linden Tree
(*Tilia cordata, T. platyphyllos*)

The heart-shaped leaves of the linden tree have always been a sure sign that it is a tree akin to the heart. "If thou lookest on the lime-leaf [linden leaf], / Thou a heart's form wilt discover; / Therefore are the lindens ever / Chosen seats of each fond lover," writes the poet Heinrich Heine

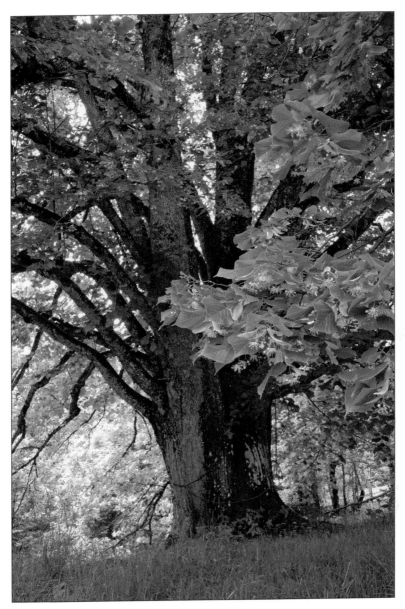

Very old blossoming linden tree (*Tilia* spp.)

in "New Spring" (Heine 1908, 190). The linden radiates joy and peace and is native to the entire Northern Hemisphere. In most areas of northern Europe, the old linden tree near the well, in the middle of the village, had not only been honored since pre-Christian times but was

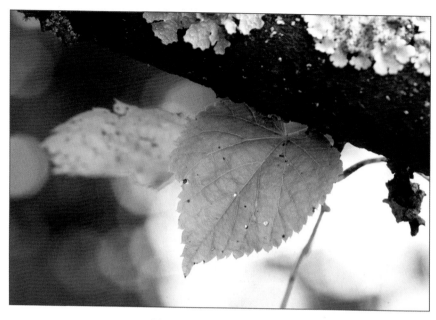

Heart-shaped linden leaf

greatly loved as well. Under its heart-shaped foliage many festivals were celebrated, such as the May dance, fairs, and weddings. In the summer, the village elders gathered in the shade of the linden to discuss important matters. Sometimes they also held the village court there.

Traditionally, the gray-haired elderly townsfolk liked to sit on a bench under the linden and dream of the hereafter. Under the bright spring greenery of the linden, young couples fell in love and dreamed about the souls of the children who might come to them from the otherworld. The famous twelfth-century traveling knight and minnesinger Walther von der Vogelweide (ca. 1170–ca. 1230) sang "Under the linden, on the heather, where the two of us had our bed." The fact that the linden tree had something to do with sensual love was well known to wise women and midwives: if one went out to gather medicinal herbs for countering a "charmed" (false) love, then the shovel or digging stick had to be made of linden wood.

In German, many folk songs still testify to the joy that can be found under the linden tree:

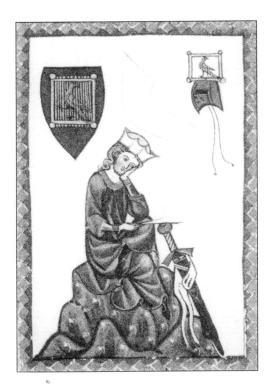

Walther von der Vogelweide (*Codex Manesse*, twelfth century)

Am Brunnen vor dem Tore, da steht ein Lindenbaum.
Ich träumt' in seinem Schatten so manchen süßen
Traum . . .

By the fountain in front of the gate there stands a
linden tree.
I've dreamed, in its shade, so many a sweet dream . . .

Or:

Kein schöner Land zu dieser Zeit als hier das unsre,
weit und breit,
wo wir uns finden wohl unter Linden zu Abendzeit.

There's no land today more beautiful than ours is, far
and wide,
Where we gather happily under lindens at eventide.

The linden tree is good for the heart; it signifies homeland, security, and peace. Martin Luther said: "If we see horsemen stopping to rest beneath the linden, it would be a sign of peace, for under the linden we drink, dance, and are merry; for the linden tree is our tree of peace and joy" (Luther 1898, 1783–84). This has always been the case. The pre-Christian Germanic peoples saw in it the presence of gentle Freya, the goddess of joy, peace, and sensuality. Freya's presence is especially felt when, at the summer solstice, the flowering linden tree is enveloped by bees seeking nectar, and the air is full of the wonderful fragrance of the blossoms and the buzzing of the bees. In classical antiquity, too, the goddess was perceived in the linden: the tree was dedicated to Aphrodite. The Scythians, a wild, horse-riding nomadic people of the southeastern European steppe, held oracles with the goddess of love under linden trees to find out information about the future.

After the religion of Peter and Paul replaced the ancient divinities like Freya, the linden tree was consecrated to Mary, Mother of God. The monks invented a pious legend that served to make the sacred tree of the heathens a blessed tree for the Christianized people as well: it was said that Jesus, sick with exhaustion, sat under a linden tree and his sufferings were lightened and he got well. So, Mary blessed the tree with fragrant blossoms. Throughout the Middle Ages, linden trees were planted next to chapels in honor of Mary, and images of the Virgin were carved from this soft sacred wood (*lignum sanctum*), whose smooth surface takes on a beautiful luster. The masterpieces of sculptors such as Tilman Riemenschneider (ca. 1460–1531), Veit Stoss (1447–1533), or Grinling Gibbons (1648–1721) were carved out of linden wood.

Linden-blossom tea is known as a sudorific tea to treat colds, not as a heart tea—it contains no cardiac glycosides or alkaloids. In cold, foggy autumn or frosty winter, when flus and colds abound, this tea, sweetened with linden-blossom honey, tastes delicious and nurtures one's health. It reminds the soul of the blissful summertime and dispels pathogenic viruses as well as melancholy thoughts. In ancient times, linden-blossom tea was used as a calmative for the nerves and heart. Recent research has confirmed that linden-blossom tea has a slightly hypotensive, anticonvulsant, and even a minimal cardiotonic effect. However, this is so small that it does not fulfill the criterion of a pharmacologically active heart remedy in the modern sense. Linden-blossom infusions are popular with people who want to achieve a calming, relaxing effect on stress-related spasms, heart pain, insomnia, and especially febrile colds (Bardeau 1993, 135).

Milk Thistle
(*Silybum marianum, Carduus marianus*)

Milk thistle, Marian thistle, or lady's thistle is a stately plant with large purple flowers and strong yellow thorns. Originally found growing from southern Europe to Asia, it is now found worldwide. In the early Middle Ages, monks from southern Europe brought it to

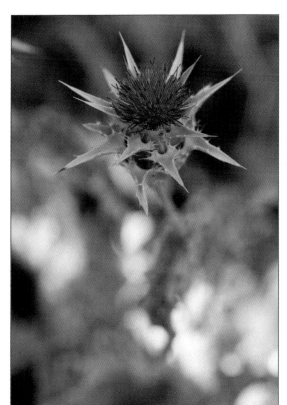

Milk thistle
(*Silybum marianum*)
blossom

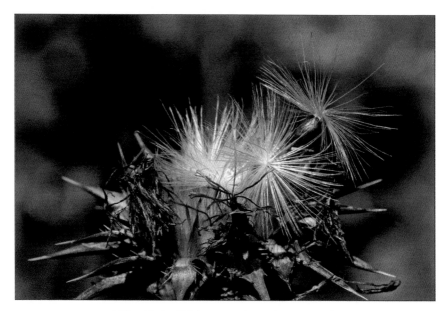

Milk thistle (*Silybum marianum*) ripe seeds

northern Europe and planted it in their monastery gardens, which were full of healing herbs. The clergymen referred to the white marbling of the leaves as the milk that fell on the plant and colored it when Mary nursed baby Jesus. Before that the Romans had said it was the milk of the goddess Hera that had marked and sanctified the plant. Milk thistle was used medicinally in a variety of ways. Dioscorides cooked the root in mead (honey wine) as an emetic. He is also said to have prescribed the plant to treat melancholia and dark moods, as did later the herbal healers of the Renaissance. But mainly—due to its signature—the prickly plant was used for stitches. Hildegard of Bingen prescribes it to alleviate "stabbing in the heart and other parts of the body." For Paracelsus, the thistle was clearly "a strong plant, indicating with its signature that hidden power is in it for healing stitches around the breast and in the sides" (Irmgard Müller 1982, 194).

Today, the seeds of milk thistle are considered a superlative liver medicine. They help with chronic liver inflammation and toxic liver damage. They are even known to be used to counter poisoning from the death cap mushroom (*Amanita phalloides*) if applied immediately.

However, this usage is relatively recent; it was not until the middle of the nineteenth century that the ingenious doctor Johannes Gottfried Rademacher announced that milk thistle–seed preparations can protect and revitalize the liver. The very bitter blessed thistle (*Cnicus benedictus*) was also believed to strengthen the heart (Ingo Müller 1993, 154).

Mullein
(*Verbascum thapsus*)

With mullein—a native of northern Europe, North Africa, and Asia and naturalized in Australia and the Americas—we encounter another plant that has been sacred since antiquity, at least in its native habitats. In the bouquet of healing and magical herbs that the women once gathered in most of Europe and took to the church for blessings on the Feast of the Assumption (August 15),* the pale-yellow flowering scepter usually stood proudly right in the middle. In the olden days throughout Europe, the felty flower stem was used as a torch after dipping it in pitch, resin, or wax. This is reflected in some of its many common names, such as hig candlewick, torches, hagtapers, witch's candle, Our Lady's candle, and tinder plant. Names alluding to its size and shape include Adam's rod and shepherd's staff, while others refer to its fuzziness: donkey's ears, hare's beard, velvet mullein, beggar's blanket, Our Lady's blanket, and felt wort. *Mullein* derives from French for "soft." It was believed to ward off fiends and witches' animals, such as rats and mice, when nailed to the barn door.

Sacred plants are typically curative. Today, we only know dried mullein flowers as an alleviating, expectorant ingredient in a tea for easing coughs. In Germany the dried, crushed leaves of this plant are

---

*The herb consecration has its origins in the Celtic harvest festival of the August full moon, which was dedicated to the hot-tempered sun god Lugus (Lugh) and his wife, the harvest goddess.

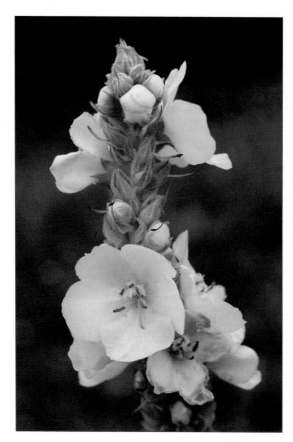

Mullein (*Verbascum thapsus*) in full blossom

also called *Takenblume* (hemorrhoid flower)* and were used to heal "swollen anal veins" (Mattioli 1563, 500). That is why the French also called the plant *herbe de saint Fiacre,* because Saint Fiacre protects against dreaded hemorrhoids, as he allegedly suffered from them himself. In Germany, mullein was dug with a piece of gold before dawn on St. John's Day (June 24) and worn on a red silk thread around the neck to protect against strokes (Paullini 1734). In Lower Bavaria, one hoped for spontaneous cures through mullein, which is there called *Himmelsbrand* (heaven's torch); sprinkled with holy water, the diseased parts of the body were touched with it and the following saying was recited:

Take is an old word for "hemorrhoid" in German.

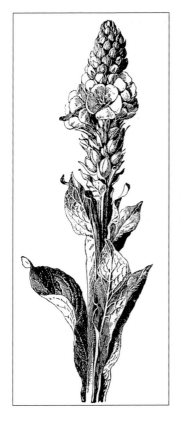

Mullein
(*Verbascum thapsus*)

Unsere Liebe Frau geht über das Land,
Sie trägt den Himmelsbrand in ihrer Hand.

Our Dear Lady travels over the land,
She carries heaven's torch in her hand.

Hildegard of Bingen wrote: "Whoever has a weak and sad heart should cook and eat the plant [she calls it *wullena**] together with meat, fish, or buns. Then his heart will be strengthened and be able to rejoice again" (Marzell 1945–1979, 232). The city doctor of Frankfurt, Adam Lonitzer (or Adamus Lonicerus), also confirmed the statement in his *Kreuterbuch,* which was first published 1557: "The common mullein

---

*"Woolen," due to the furry leaves.

weed, with other herbs in the stew of meat, or especially cooked with other vegetables, cures all the diseases of the heart" (Lonicerus 1679, 314). The plant also confers courage: "He who carries the stalk with him has no fear, and no harm will come to him," states the fifteenth-century handwritten *Herbarium* of Pseudo-Apuleius (Marzell 1938, 231).

Oregano
(*Origanum vulgare*)

This red-flowered, fragrant plant—which in German is also called *Wohlgemuth* (cheerful)—from the mint family has an antispasmodic, stomach-strengthening, cough-soothing, nerve-strengthening, and warming effect. Originally native to the Mediterranean Basin, it quickly

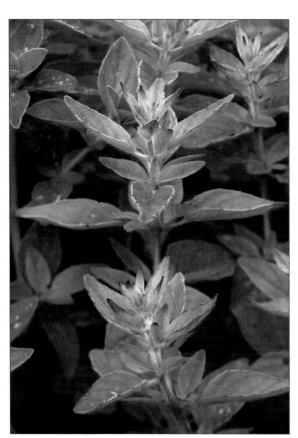

Oregano
(*Origanum vulgare*)
leaves before
blossoming

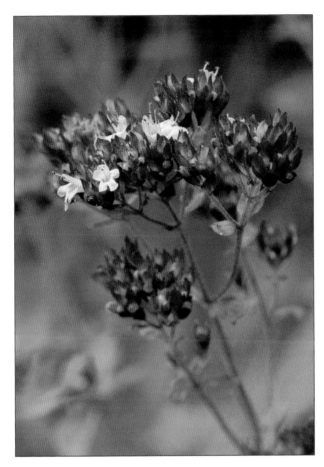

Oregano
(*Origanum vulgare*)
blossom

naturalized in the temperate Northern Hermisphere. It contains essential oil (thymol, carvacrol) as well as bitter substances and tannins. The pretty herb was added to bathwater to strengthen the nerves. It was used in women's baths as well as in the sachets of dried herbs that were traditionally placed in the bed during childbirth to soothe mother and newborn. Other herbs in the sachet were cleavers (also called bedstraw), thyme, sweetgrass, chamomile, lavender, and various others. Also called wild marjoram, the plant was believed to protect against demons and evil sorcery and to give courage—a trait of the heart. A devil who was after a girl, but found out that she was carrying a bouquet of wild marjoram, uttered this curse:

Roter Dost!
Hätt' ich das gewost,
Hätt' ich das vernomme,
Wär ich net daher gekomme.

Red marjoram!
If that I'd known,
If that I'd sensed,
I wouldn't have gone after her.

And another devil, who wanted to accost a woman in a beer cellar, cried out angrily:

Hättest du nicht Dorant und Dosten,
Tät's dich dein Leben kosten!

If you wouldn't have had horehound and marjoram,
It would have cost you your life!

Raspberry
(*Rubus idaeus*)

In his 1663 treatise *Parnassus medicinalis,* the Ulm physician Johann Joachim Becher writes that raspberries cheer the heart:

Hindbeeren geben den Brombeeren nicht viel nach,
Sie stillen von der Ruhr im Leib das Ungemach.
Vor andrem stehen sie dem Herzen treulich bey
Durch Kunst darauß man macht und nützet dreyerlei:
Den Durst sie löschen tun der Essig, Syrup, Safft;
Dem matten Hertzen sie verleyhen große Krafft.
(Marzell 2002, 101)

Raspberries are truly not inferior to blackberries,
They stifle the misfortune of dysentry in the body.

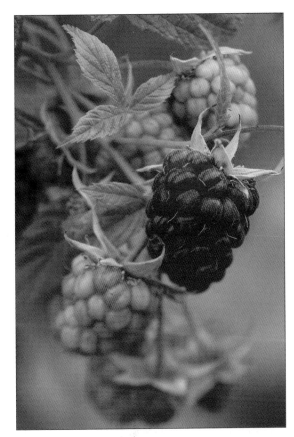

Raspberry
(*Rubus idaeus*)
fruit

They are, in particular, faithful to the heart
Artfully, they are prepared and used for three things:
Quenching thirst as vinegar, syrup, or juice;
To the tired heart, they lend great strength.

"Nowadays, hardly anything is known about the 'heart-strengthening' properties of raspberries," laments Heinrich Marzell (2002, 101). The German word for the berry is *Himbeere,* which modern speakers of the language might assume refers to a "heaven berry" (with the first element a clipped form of *Himmel,* "heaven"), especially in light of how delicious these berries are. However, they would be mistaken; the name comes from an earlier form, *Hindbeere,* which refers to a berry that young female deer (hind) like to eat, thus a "hind berry." The gentler

Himbeere, or "hind berry" is, the West Germanic peoples believed, the wife of the *Hirschbeere,* or "stag berry"—that is, the blackberry (Marzell 2002, 102). In the symbolic imagination of heathen Europe, the deer was also seen as the embodiment of the sun spirit. Starting in the spring, the sun leaps across the sky over the course of the year like a stag. Plants dedicated to the hind are those in harmony with the sun stag. They are also referred to as "brides of the sun" (*Sonnebräute*). They bring humans into harmony with the natural internal and external rhythms. Red raspberry is native to Europe and northern Asia, but it is now grown worldwide.

Rose
(*Rosa* spp.)

The sweetly scented rose appeals to the soul, the heart, the innermost part of a person. Originally, all roses were wild and grew in Europe, North America, northwest Africa, and many parts of Asia and Oceania. In modern times, the cultivars are known worldwide. The

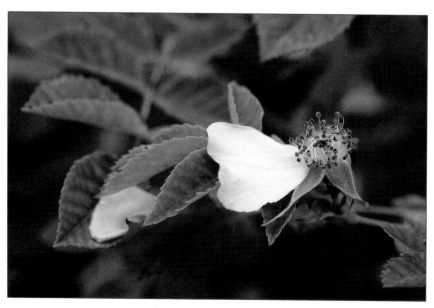

Rose (*Rosa* spp.), last remaining petal

individual petals are heart shaped, and the color is crimson. When a man gives a red rose to his beloved, he gives her his heart. Yes, the person dearest to one's heart is indeed a rose: "A rose by any other name would smell as sweet," says Juliet of Romeo. Or, as a German folksong goes:

> *Als ich im Gärtlein war,*
> *Nahm ich ein Blümlein wahr,*
> *Brach mir ein Röselein,*
> *das soll mein eigen sein.*

> When I was in the garden,
> I saw a flower,
> I plucked a precious rose blossom,
> to have as my very own.

People have always been convinced that love, even sensual love, resides in the heart. In antiquity, the rose was the flower of the goddess of love, Venus or Aphrodite. Also bedecked with roses were Hebe, the goddess of youth; Ganymede, the cupbearer of the gods, who brings them intoxicating wine; Erato, the Muse of love poetry; and the lusty, drunken Dionysus. Even in the Islamic culture, especially among the Sufis, the rose is associated with the mystery of love—the soul opens to love like a blossoming rose. For the more orthodox Muslims, the rose symbolizes the blood of the Prophet and his two grandsons, Hasan and Husayn.

Among the Germanic peoples, the rose—along with sloe, hawthorn, blackberry, and other thorny plants—was a component of the impenetrable hedge that protected cultivated land, meadows, fields, and the homestead in the middle, separating them from the wilderness. The open hearth, where these people from the cold, northern lands warmed themselves and were cheered by its beautiful light, was the heart of each dwelling and also of the settlement. Humans and animals could sleep peacefully surrounded by this thorny hedge. Any kind of enemy feared

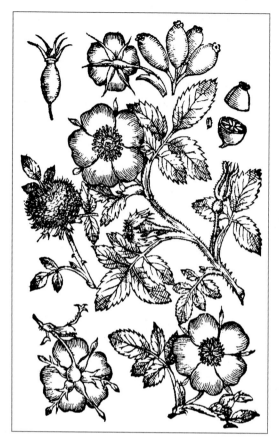

The wild rose

the thorns of the hedge-brush. The red rose hips ripening in the fall were believed to protect not only against wicked spells but also from lightning and thunder. It was long held that when a werewolf encounters a rose, it loses its coat of fur and becomes human again (Gallwitz 1992, 205).

For Christians, the rose is the symbol of Mary. The five petals stand for the five wounds of the Savior who redeemed the world. Walafrid Strabo (808–849), the cross-eyed monk in the Reichenau Monastery (on an island in Lake Constance), recognized in the rose a symbol of the Passion, for its color is that of blood and its blossom a heart wound (Stoffler 2002, 131). But also the purity of the Mother of God is reflected in the rose. In old paintings Mary is often depicted surrounded by roses. Among those who are blessed, the Immaculate Virgin rests on a throne in a rose arbor in the heart, similarly to how in South Asia the goddess has her place upon a lotus flower.

One can certainly expect strong healing powers from such a symbolic, sacred plant. In the medieval humoral theory, the rose is considered cool and dry; protects against poison; strengthens the heart, brain, spirit, stomach, liver, and spleen; and takes anger away from the soul by purging yellow bile (Ingo Müller 1993, 205). Rose oil helps when the heart is disturbed by sadness, anxiety, worry, grief, disappointment, discouragement, lovesickness, hurt feelings, anger, or isolation (Keller 1999, 121).

Rosemary
(*Salvia rosmarinus*)

Rosemary is a native of the Mediterranean Basin, but it is now cultivated worldwide. In the eighth century Benedictine monks brought the plant over the Alps into northern Europe. Contrary to what one might think, rosemary has nothing to do with either roses or Mary—the name comes from the Latin *ros maris,* meaning "dewdrops of the sea." This, in turn, refers to the love goddess Aphrodite, who was born out of sea foam. Rosemary is suggestive of sensual love and its counterpart, death. Both are matters of the heart. Otto Brunfels described the virtues of the distilled water of this aromatic member of the Lamiaceae family in his work *Contrafayt Kreuterbuch* (Straßburg, 1532) as follows:

> *Stercket die Memory, das ist die gedächtnüsß.*
> *Behütet vor der pestilentz,*
> *erwörmet das marck in den beynen.*
> *Bringet die sprach härwider.*
> *Macht keck und hertzhafftig,*
> *macht jung geschaffen,*
> *retardiert das Alter, so man es allen tag trincket,*
> *ist ein theriacks für alles gyfft . . .*

[It] strengthens the memory—that is, the recollection.
Protects against the pestilence,
warms the marrow in the bones.
Restores speech.
Makes one bold and hearty,
keeps one young,
retards old age, so if one drinks it every day,
it is a theriac (antidote) for any poison . . .

In *Hamlet*, Shakespeare has Ophelia say: "There's rosemary, that's for remembrance." Brunfels also wrote that the herb is suitable for promoting sensual desire. This is reflected in a German nursery rhyme as well:

Rosmarin und Thymian
Wächst in unserem Garten,
Unser Annchen is die Braut,
kann nicht länger warten.

Rosemary and thyme
grow near the garden gate,
Our Annie is the bride,
and can hardly wait.

The Straßburg surgeon Walther Ryff (1500–1548) explicitly mentions rosemary wine as a heart remedy: "The spirits of the heart and of the entire body experience joy through this drink, which dispels despondency and worries." The herbalist pastor Kneipp agrees: "Rosemary wine, drunk in small portions, has proved itself to be an outstanding remedy for heart ailments. It has a calming effect and, in the case of dropsy of the heart, boosts excretion via the urine" (Kneipp 1894, 145).

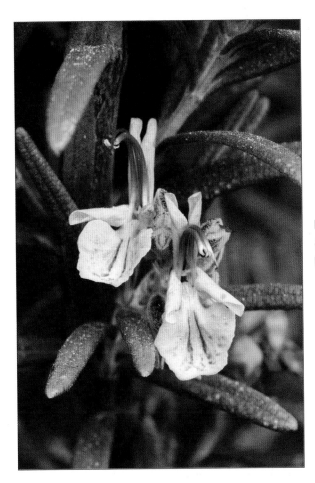

Rosemary
(*Salvia rosmarinus*)
leaves and blossoms

Modern research confirms these observations. German phytotherapist Ursel Bühring writes:

> Rosemary stimulates the blood circulation and thus also the blood
> circulation of the brain. . . . In addition, rosemary increases the coro-
> nary flow—that is, it supports the circulation of the coronary vessels
> and thus the heart activity. Rosemary promotes blood circulation
> to the extremities, which warms the limbs and is beneficial for the
> condition of cold hands and feet, which frequently accompanies low
> blood pressure. (Bühring 2007, 213)

Speedwell
(*Veronica officinalis*)

Speedwell was dedicated to Saint Veronica. She is said to have handed her veil to Jesus to wipe the sweat from his brow as he was being driven through the narrow streets of Jerusalem, carrying the cross upon which he would be crucified. This legend points to the sudorific, blood-cleansing effect of the plant. As Hieronymus Bock said, the plant is an "excellently reliable medicine for all poisonous, pestilent fevers," for "these must flee the heart and be sweated out"; the old master of herbalogy further noted that it was "quite a good plant for a malicious spleen" (Marzell 1938, 234). According to the old theory of humoral medicine, the spleen was the organ of dark and heavy Saturn; thus, if the spleen is ill, black bile rises from it and can make the heart heavy and melancholy.

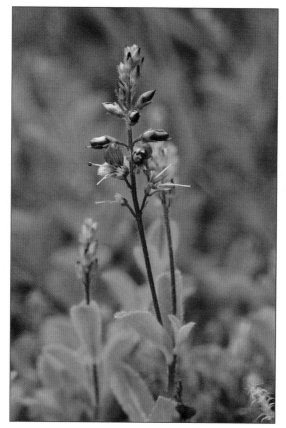

Speedwell
(*Veronica officinalis*)
leaves and blossoms

Speedwell was taken as tea to alleviate various sufferings and ailments. The sixteenth-century German botanist Leonhart Fuchs called the herb *Grundheil* (a basic healer). In Hamburg, it was called *sta up an ga weg* (stand up and walk), which refers to the words of Christ when he told a paralyzed man he was healed (Matthew 9:5–6). Elsewhere in Germany it was known as *Trost aller Welt* (universal consolation), *Allerweltsheil* (world's salvation), *Heil aller Schmerzen* (easer of all pain), and *Zuhause ist er nicht* ("He's not at home," a reference to the fever-spirit seeking to attack the patient). The tea was used for blood purification (as the herbalist pastor Kneipp and Maria Treben indicate) and as a stomach, liver, lung, and spleen healer. Speedwell tea was also considered healing for nervousness, mental exhaustion, dizziness, and melancholia. Anyone who is brokenhearted can drink the juice of the plant and should be cured soon (Gallwitz 1992, 109).

St. John's Wort
(*Hypericum perforatum*)

The flowers of St. John's wort, which blooms at midsummer, look like swirling light chakras. If you squeeze them, a red juice comes out: the blood of Saint John. In older times the juice was believed to have sprung from the blood of the sun god Baldur, fatally wounded at the summer solstice, or—as the Christians believed—from the blood of the beheaded John the Baptist. Either way, it is self-evident that St. John's wort, which is native to Eurasia, has long played a part in the summer solstice festivals of Europe. It is a sacred, salubrious plant. It drives off the evil spirits of darkness. As Paracelsus said, it chases away *phantasmata,* or pathological illusions, "diseases without corpus and substance" (Pörksen 1988, 78). It brings sunlight into the heart and disperses the heavy dark clouds of melancholia and *Schwarzesehen* (pessimism). It was also used as an incense to ward off dangerous storms and to protect the farmstead from lightning and the ripening grainfields from hail. This is evident in an old German saying:

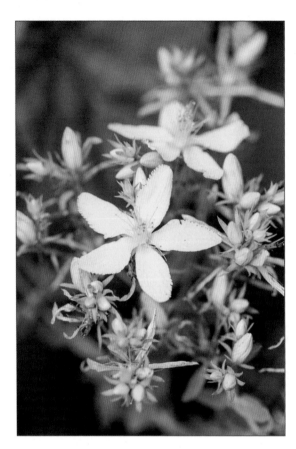

St. John's wort
(*Hypericum perforatum*)
in full bloom

Eisenhart und Hartenau,
Brennt's an, damit das Gewitter stau!

Eisenhart [vervain] and *Hartenau* [St. John's wort],
Smudge with them to stop the thunderstorm!

Traditionally, children's bedrooms and sanatoria were censed with the dried plant; it was stuck in the four corners of the house or field; it was put into a child's first bath; braided into the first sheaf of grain that was cut at harvesttime; or a bit of it was mixed into the hay of bewitched cattle.* It was also believed that "such a man that has lost his

---

*If the cattle weren't producing as much milk as normal, or otherwise seemed a bit sick, it was usually blamed on some kind of witchcraft.

senses by enchanting love and turned into a fool"—that is, a victim of a love spell—could be brought back to his senses and spared from heart-break by drinking St. John's wort wine or wearing an amulet made from the plant (Hildegard of Bingen 1957). For good reason the plant was called names like devil chase and scare devil (*fuga daemonum*). Even the Dominican inquisitors gave the so-called witches on the torture rack St. John's wort tea to sip because it is supposed to dissolve pacts with the devil. For they knew as well:

> *Dost, Hartheu und Wegscheid*
> *Thun dem Teuffel viel Leidt.*

> *Dost* [oregano], *Hartheu* [St. John's wort], *and*
> *Wegscheid* [chicory]
> Do the devil a lot of harm.

(It probably would have been better if the inquisitors drank the tea themselves.)

In his *Buch der Natur* (Book of Nature), Konrad von Megenberg (1309–1374) tells us that "the herb strengthens the heart and liver, cleanses the kidneys, and heals ulcers." Indeed, St. John's wort is good for our heart; it has a calming effect on our psyche. It brings light to the soul and gives us happy, vivid dreams. Anyone who drinks the tea and then observes the psychosomatic effect can sense this. Meanwhile, clinical studies have shown that St. John's wort contains synergistic active complexes. These include flavonoids (quercetin, quercitrin), which act as a mono-amino oxidase inhibitor (MAOI) and stop the breakdown (reabsorption) of the three major neurotransmitters: sero-tonin (the happiness hormone), noradrenaline, and dopamine. These neurotransmitters occupy the receptors for calming signals (Phaneuf 2005, 289). The light-mediating (photosensitizing) red dye hypericin inhibits depression by also activating the brain's neurotransmitter bal-ance. In addition, St. John's wort reduces the stress hormones cortico-tropin (or adrenocorticotropic hormone, ACTH) and corticosterone produced in the adrenal glands. It even contains melatonin, which has a harmonizing effect on the pineal gland.* In addition, the plant activates the tranquilizer GABA (gamma-aminobutyric acid) in the brain. There are also tannins that increase heart circulation and essential oils that alleviate pain (Bäumler 2007, 222).

St. John's wort has no serious adverse health effects or side effects. It works cumulatively—that is, the mood-enhancing effect occurs gradually after three weeks of regular use. Incidentally, it is interesting that St. John's wort accelerates the reversal of chemical-pharmaceutical foreign substances in the body. It makes some unnatural (chemical) medicines less effective, as observed in the following (Phaneuf 2005, 291):

- anticoagulatory blood thinners such as phenprocoumon (Marcoumar, Marcumar, Falithrom) and warfarin (Coumadin), which are used in cases at risk for thrombosis, pulmonary embolism, and myocardial infarction
- blood lipids such as simvastatin (Zocor)
- immunosuppressants such as cyclosporin and tacrolimus (also known as fujimycin, or FK-506), on which those with organ transplants are dependent
- synthetic cardiac-output-enhancing agents such as digoxin (Lanoxin) and theophylline (also known as 1,3-dimethylxanthine)
- psychotropic drugs such as amitriptyline (Elavil†)
- antihistamines such as fexofenadine (Allegra and FX 24)
- virus inhibitors like indinavir (IDV, Crixivan) and nevirapine (NVP, Viramune), which are prescribed for those with HIV infections
- methadone (Dolophine) for heroin addicts
- midazolam (Versed), which is used for anesthesia and sedation

---

*The pineal gland, or epiphysis, absorbs cosmic light stimuli and brings the organism in sync with the natural day-night rhythm and the lunar rhythms.
†Elavil was taken off the market by the FDA in 2006, but the generic form, amitriptyline, is still available.

◆ the chemotherapeutic cancer drug irinotecan (Camptosar), which also exits the body sooner than desired during the therapy when St. John's wort is taken simultaneously

The effect of birth control pills can also be shut down by this sun plant. Despite the pill, time and again "St. John's wort babies" are born—and about which the parents, despite whatever previous reservations they may have had, are usually very happy.

St. John's wort primarily stimulates the production of a liver enzyme (cytochrome P450 3A4) that accelerates the detoxification and excretion of foreign chemical substances and in this way weakens the effects of many pharmaceutical drugs. This power of St. John's wort is considered to be highly problematic in today's medical world, and there are loud voices that seek to prohibit the light-transmitting, mood-enhancing, demon-repelling herb by law.

But St. John's wort—which joins the soul with the sunlight, with the radiance and the pulse of the cosmic heart—brings us back into harmony with all living things.

Storksbill
(*Geranium robertianum*)

The stinking storksbill, also known as herb Robert or stinking Bob, which grows along the edges of woodlands and between pavement cracks in the cities—with its seeds carried there by ants—is primarily used as an astringent, hemostatic healing herb for wounds and cuts. It is a native of Europe, North Africa, and parts of Asia and has become an invasive plant in North America (in the English-speaking world, the storksbill/geranium genus is commonly called cranesbill). The Swiss herbalist pastor Johann Künzle called it an "herb of God's grace" and prescribed it boiled in red wine for gastrointestinal inflammation and as a tea for kidney and stomach pain, sore throat, and tumors of the gums. He recommended poultices made from the soaked dry herb to relieve eczema and rashes (Künzle 2008). In traditional folk medicine, the

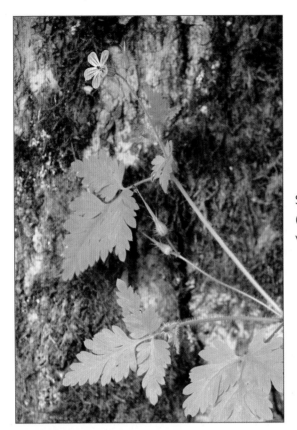

Storksbill
(*Geranium robertianum*)
whole plant

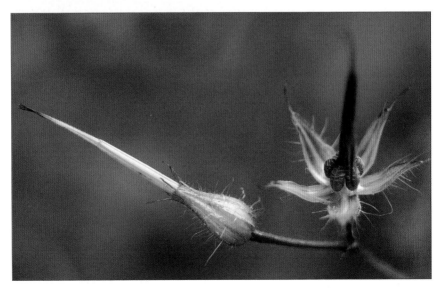

Storksbill (*Geranium robertianum*) unripe and ripe seed

fresh juice was used for the external treatment of skin diseases, ulcers, wounds, erysipelas, and nerve inflammations, or added as a decoction to the bath.

In even earlier times, storksbill was also used to strengthen the heart. In her *Liber simplicis medicinae,* Hildegard of Bingen recommended a powder made from storksbill (*storkensnauel*) with other plants:*

> Those who have heart complaints and are always saddened should take storksbill and, to a lesser extent, pennyroyal (*Mentha pulegium*), and rue to a lesser extent than pennyroyal, pulverize everything and eat this powder often with bread. The heart will be strengthened and become joyful, for the cold of storksbill, mixed with the heat of pennyroyal and rue, as well as the bread's strength, will lead the corrupted warm and cold juices that damage the human heart back to a healthy state. (Hildegard of Bingen 2010, 142)

Another Hildegard recipe that works against "love enchantment and magic spells"; makes one healthy; and gives courage, strength, and luck consists of pulverized storksbill root, mallow, and plantain. It is sufficient to just carry this powder in a satchel (Gallwitz 1992, 225). The herbal doctor Adamus Lonicerus (Lonitzer) confirms this statement: "Whoever is feeling bad / and would be sad / should use the herb with pennyroyal and rue / each equally / powdered / and eaten with bread / strengthens the heart and makes it joyful" (Lonicerus 1679, 348). Paracelsus also mentioned that the chopped or powdered herb on buttered bread is a good remedy for the attack of "black bile," which can afflict the heart.

Perhaps this superstition also has an empirical basis, for the essential oils of the related rose geranium (*Perlagonium graveolens*), originally from South Africa, are said to have a balancing—simultaneously stimulating and calming—effect on the mind. The rose-like scent of this

---

*Scholars are not entirely sure if the *storkensnauel* to which Hildegard refers is the *Geranium pratense* or the *Geranium robertianum* (herb Robert). Most—including this author—agree that the latter is meant, because it is more common and prefers growing near human habitation.

geranium is a preferred medium, especially with matters of the heart and for a state of vulnerability (Keller 1999, 105).

Storksbill was also important for another matter of the heart: the herb was placed under the bed when a couple wanted to signal to forefathers, the ancestors (from whom children were believed to come), that they were ready to welcome a baby. The plant has, with its red "legs" and a seed capsule that looks like the head and bill of this bird, the signature of the stork, the child-bringer Adebar.* In many places in Europe, the stork, a sacred bird of the Great Goddess, is believed to bring the children's souls from the otherworld. It is considered a sign of good luck if a stork pair builds a nest on the roof of a house. (In Central Europe, one may even see a stork painted on the door, or a replica hanging on the roof when a new baby is in the house.) The name herb Robert refers to Saint Ruprecht or Robert (died 715 CE), an Iro-Scottish missionary, the apostle to the Bavarians and the first bishop of Salzburg, considered by some folklorists to have replaced Donar (Thor) as the protector of marriage and the household (Carl 1957, 107).

Strawberry, Wild
(*Fragaria vesca*)

The wild strawberry, the first sweet and delicious fruit of the year, brings joy to everyone and pleases the child in us. It grows naturally throughout most of the Northern Hemisphere. Like the fragrant violet or the delicate daisies, this little rose plant has always been considered a sign of the eternally returning goddess of nature, Freya, the mistress of the joy of life. For the Christians, this thornless plant of the rose family, which has a sweet fruit without a hard shell or pit, became the symbol of Mary. A folk legend tells that Mary leads the children's souls in paradise out to a meadow full of strawberries.

---

*Adebar, "bringer of good fortune, luck," fom the Old High German *Odobero* (bringer of good) is an old name for the stork (*Storch*). He brings the children from a swamp or out of a deep well—in other words, from the realm of Frau Holle (Mother Holda).

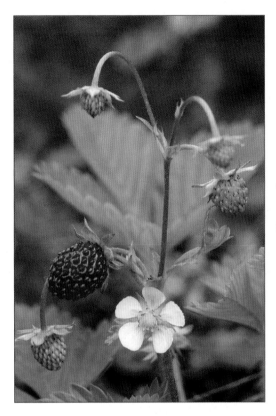

Wild strawberry
(*Fragaria vesca*)
blossom and fruit

Valerian
(*Valeriana officinalis*)

Elderly ladies in the Victorian era took a few drops of valerian tincture to soothe their nerves and hearts. These drops helped them cope with too much excitement and allowed them to sleep better and no longer be plagued by nocturnal heart palpitations. Valerian is not a real heart remedy in the modern sense. Rather, it helps calm the nerves when they are under continual stress. It is a native of Europe and Asia.

It is interesting to note that valerian has been known since antiquity and was traded in pharmacies—hence the byname *officinalis*.* But it was not until the industrial age that the medicinal plant was discovered as

---

*The medieval Latin word *officina* referred to the salesroom and workshop (recipe area) of the pharmacy.

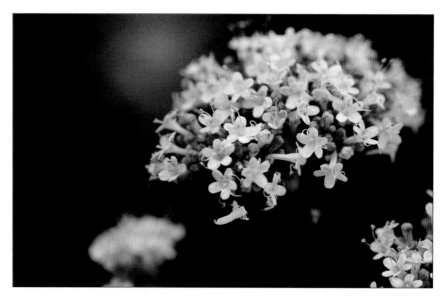

Valerian (*Valeriana officinalis*) in full bloom

a nerve remedy; the English doctor John Hill discovered its application in this regard in the latter part of the eighteenth century. Christoph Wilhelm Hufeland, the ingenious German doctor from the Goethe era (1770–1830), praised it as "one of the best nerve remedies" when taken as tea in the mornings and evenings. He witnessed how "long-time nerve damage, hysteria, and convulsions of all kinds disappeared." Since then, the root has been prepared as a pill, a tincture, in wine, as a bath additive, or as a cold-water extract (eight hours) to relieve all kinds of tension and excited states, sleep disorders, depression, vegetative dystonia, cardiac neuroses, circulatory problems, and mental exhaustion. Valerian has an adaptogenic effect—that is, it stabilizes the patient. It can calm the restless, but also stimulate those who are exhausted. It does not narcoticize, confuse the senses, or make one tired, but it provides a person who is highly stressed with sufficient relaxation that he or she may fall asleep. And those who do not need sleep can easily read a book or drive a car. Contrary to what is sometimes claimed, valerian is not addictive.

Before the Industrial Revolution, the plant was known as an aphrodisiac, an eye cure, and a safeguard against the plague and the wickedness of witches and devils. The aphrodisiac property of the beautiful pink flowering woodland herb was mentioned in an old manuscript from Castle Wolfsthurn (fifteenth century): "If you want to make good friendship among men and women, then take Valerianam (roots) and mash them and give it to them to drink in wine" (Marzell 2002, 255). The venerable herbalist Otto Brunfels (sixteenth century) affirmed that Valerian makes "blissful, united and frivolous, where two drink of its water" (Marzell 2002, 255). An old superstition claims: "If you put valerian in your mouth and kiss someone, you win that person over." Or the age-old advice to a horny man: so that women cannot deny him anything, he should carry valerian and silver thistle root in the pocket of his pants.

One might think that the alleged aphrodisiac effect of valerian is because cats react wildly to the smell of valerian. After all, cats are a symbol of eroticism and companions of the goddesses of love.* Valerian's pheromone-like odor (isovaleric acid) resembles that of a man's underarm perspiration—which is purported to have a subliminal sexual signal effect. But valerian is probably also an erotic elixir, because when it is steeped in wine it has a relaxing effect, which is conducive to amorous love play. In earlier times St. George's Day (April 23) was considered the best day to dig the root. The day of the knight George—who stabs the earth dragon with his lance and liberates the virgin whom it held captive—is a good day for love magic. It is said that on this day infertile women can be made fertile. Medieval Christians called it *Sancti Georgii herba,* which remains one of its common names in English: St. George's herb.

The relaxing effect of valerian also partly explains its use as an eye medicine. The botanist Leonhart Fuchs wrote: "A few drops of valerian root that has been boiled in wine or water and dropped into the eyes clears the vision" (Fuchs 1543). It was one of the goldsmith's secrets to make such eye water when they had to do very fine work.

---

*During the Soviet occupation of Latvia, schoolchildren and various delegations were obliged to visit the Lenin Statue in Riga. Dissidents smeared valerian juice on the base of the statue to attract tomcats. The statue smelled so awful from all the pissing and spraying that most visitors would not stay long.

In Transylvania, infirm eyes were traditionally treated by the healer chewing valerian root and then breathing his breath onto the eyes. And in St. Gallen (Switzerland), the root was part of the *Augebündeli* (eye bundle), a sachet that was worn around the neck to alleviate inflamed eyes.

Furthermore, it was believed that valerian was able to keep away pestilence, witches, and devils. More specifically, "witches" and "devils" can be seen as representing cramped, hardened, tense, dissatisfied, and unhappy souls who are incapable of allowing others any sort of joy. No wonder valerian can help. Many such stories can be found in the folklore, such as this one from Mecklenburg:

A boy went to gather nuts in the forest one Sunday morning. Suddenly, a forest devil stood in front of him. But he could not harm the boy, because by chance some valerian had stuck to the child's shoes. Outraged, the devil cried:

"*Harrst du nich Bullerjan,*
Ick wull mit die Noetplücken gan,
Dat di dei Ogen sulln in'n Nacken stan."

"If you didn't have valerian,
I'd have like to go nut-picking with you,
until your eyes were on your neck!"

(That is, the devil would have twisted and broken his neck.)

The magical herb also drives away witches, as is clear from the following saying: *Baldrian, Dost und Dill, die Hex' kann nicht wie sie will!* (Valerian, oregano, and dill—the witch cannot do as she will!). A sprig of valerian hanging above the door prevents witches from entering a house or stable. If the farmer places valerian in the drinking trough, his cattle cannot be bewitched (causing their milk to dry up, for example, or a sickness to befall them). And if a bouquet of valerian is hung from the ceiling of a room, whenever a witch enters, the bouquet—called bustle (*Unruh*) because it is always in motion—will suddenly stop.

Valerian can even keep away envious elves. In Sweden, where the plant is called *Velandsört* (Wieland's root), the young groom should always bring some valerian root into the bridal chamber because the elves are often jealous of happy young lovers. The name suggests that valerian was used to conjure up a lot of magic: the magical blacksmith Wieland (English Wayland; Old Norse Velent), who appears in many Germanic legends, is known to be a sorcerer.

Valerian is repeatedly mentioned as a protection against or cure for the plague. When the Black Death raged in Germany in the mid-fourteenth century and people were at their wits' end, a forest lady appeared, a friendly spirit of the woods, and said:

> *Esst Bibernell und Baldrian,*
> *so geht die Pest euch nichts an.*

> Eat burnet and valerian,
> And the plague will pass you by.

In West Saxony, a gnome-like little gray man appeared and went from house to house knocking on the door. For each knock he made on the door, someone died in the house. But he said to one man and his wife: "Your neighbors are going to die; you will have to bury them. If you drink valerian, then you will be spared" (Schrödter 1997, 213). In Silesia, a spirit told the frightened people: "Cook, cook valerian. It will soon be better again!" (*Koch, koch Baldrian. Es wird schon wieder besser wa'n!*).

Valerian was of great benefit in other ways. It was placed under the pillows of toddlers when they suffered from seizures. It was put in beehives to keep the bees healthy and protect them from robber bees. Pharmacists stirred valerian into theriac, the cure-all remedy of antiquity. Executioners chewed valerian root to keep them calm during their gruesome work. Keen fishermen still bathe their worms in valerian juice to lure the fish, especially trout. Biodynamic gardeners and farmers spray the compost with valerian juice (Biodynamic Preparation 507) to make the humus receptive to the beneficial influences of Saturn and other cosmic archetypes. Valerian preparation is also sprayed on tomatoes to make them more frost resistant. And it is not only cats that are attracted to valerian; rats are claimed to be as well. This is how the Pied Piper of Hamelin is said to have been able to lead the rats out of town.

Valerian does not contain cardiac glycosides, but it does contain a mixture of different drug complexes that in isolation are relatively ineffective. Among them are valepotriates, which inhibit the breakdown of GABA (gamma-aminobutyric acid), a chemical messenger in the brain—a lack of GABA is associated with stress, nervousness, and anxiety. Added to this are essential oils and valeric acid, which, when combined, soothe the beta waves in the brain in favor of the slower delta and theta waves. Among other things, it also contains the alkaloids chatinin and valerin, which relax the digestive system. The great German phytotherapist Dr. Rudolf Fritz Weiss explained that valerian has proved to be a prime example of the fact that, although no single active substance can be found, the interaction of different substances results in the therapeutic effect (Weiss 2001, 50).

Vervain
(*Verbena officinalis*)

Courage has its seat in the heart. Courage is a heart virtue (Old French *corage,* from the Latin *cor,* "heart"), and hardly any plant supports a courageous heart more than vervain, a native plant of Europe, also known as verbena. Even among the Romans, verbena was considered a diplomat's and envoy's herb because the ambassadors wore it when they negotiated with enemies. The herald or ambassador was called a *verbenarius,* and peace treaties were touched with vervain stalks to ratify them. Pliny reports that the council of priests, which was responsible for war and peace, wore crowns of the sacred plant (*herba sacra*). The Gallic Druids wore plaited verbena wreaths around their heads to protect themselves from enchantment by magical songs. They also

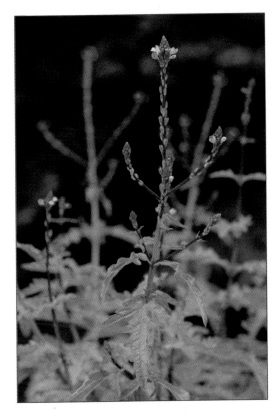

Vervain (*Verbena officinalis*) leaves and blossoms

used the plant for fortune-telling, but the Roman judge Pliny dismissed such beliefs, saying: "The Magi [Druidic magicians] especially make the maddest statements about the plant" (Pliny 1966, 215).

Since the Celtic Iron Age, vervain was the herb of the blacksmiths and considered a sacred plant. Smiths were believed to be sorcerers who dared to wrest their metal embryos from the earth and then make them glow in fire and pound them on the anvil with heavy hammers. The blacksmith had to fear the revenge of the Earth Mother and the earth dragon for this outrage, but the vervain plant protected him. The altars of the lightning- and thunder-god Jupiter, the natural enemy of the earth dragon, were also swept with vervain stalks. Later in the European Middle Ages, the knights rubbed their iron weapons with the herb and wore it as an amulet. Vervain was also used as a healing plant for wounds made by iron weapons. Treasure hunters who went out digging on the night of the iron-armored knight, St. George (April 23), wore vervain as a precaution to protect them from the earth dragon.

Olaf Rippe, a practitioner who knows how to make Paracelsus's medical suggestions palatable for modern people, says that this plant can still be used to strengthen courage. During visits to the authorities, salary negotiations, or examinations, a protective amulet or a few drops of vervain tincture helps to create the necessary serenity and strengthens self-confidence (Rippe 2005, 120). Vervain belongs not only to the planet Mars but also to his beloved Venus. As everyone knows, the heart is not only the abode of boldness but also of love. Many a love spell has made use of this herb. The early Swiss scientist, doctor, and alchemist Leonhard Thurneysser (1531–1596) gave the following advice to love-hungry men:

> *Verbeen, Agrimonia, Modelgeer,*
> *Karfreitags graben hilft dir sehr,*
> *dass dir die Frauen werden hold.*
> *Doch brauch kein Eisen, grab's mit Gold!*

> Verbena, agrimony, gentian,
> Good Friday's digging will be of great help,
> So the ladies will be devoted to you.
> But don't use iron, dig with gold!

Vervain, which contains iridioglycosides such as verbenalin and hastatoside, as well as tannins and bitter substances, has a broad range of efficacy. An overactive thyroid gland makes the heart beat faster (heart palpitations) and blood pressure increases. Vervain tea or a cold-water extract can help with such nervous and functional heart problems because it has a calming and regulating effect on the thyroid gland. In addition, vervain is slightly astringent, anti-inflammatory, uterine-contracting (caution during pregnancy!), secretionary, a galactagogue, metabolism-stimulating, sleep-promoting, and calmative during menopause. As a Bach flower remedy, vervain is claimed to help the exhausted personalities who do not give up easily to regain their strength.

The bitter-tasting, native European vervain is not identical to the lemon-scented verbena tea that can be bought in supermarkets. The latter plant (*Lippia citriodora*) comes from South America and grows in the Mediterranean as an invasive species.

Woodruff
(*Asperula odorata, Galium odoratum*)

Woodruff is a Eurasian native, found in temperate zones. In Germany, one of the many common names of woodruff is *Herzfreund* (heart's friend), because, as Tabernaemontanus wrote: "It should also strengthen and delight the heart" (Tabernaemontanus 1588–1591). Woodruff, a member of the madder family (Rubiaceae), blossoms in May, and in Germany it is a favorite ingredient in the May bowl punch (*Maitrank* or *Maibowle*) made at that time of year. As early as 854, the Benedictine monk Wandalbert is reported to have said:

> *Schütte perlenden Wein*
> *auf das Waldmeisterlein.*
>
> Pour sparkling wine
> on the beloved woodruff.

Hieronymus Bock, who called Woodruff "liver plant," wrote: "If one puts this beloved plant and its blossom in wine and drinks of it, one feels a gaiety, and from it we gain a healthy liver" (Bock 1539). The herb must be allowed to wilt for a couple of days to develop the coumarin-based aroma. Then it is steeped in white wine (possibly with a little lemon, sugar, and some ground ivy and black currant leaves) for several hours, and an equal amount of champagne is added just before serving. The potion has a relaxing and slightly aphrodisiac effect. It was probably part of the Celtic May Festival, when the flower-adorned goddess

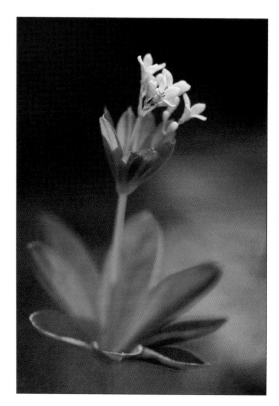

Woodruff
(*Galium odoratum*)

of plants wedded the sun god Bel, at which time Maypoles were erected and the wedding of the gods was exuberantly celebrated.

As a tea, woodruff has an antiseptic effect; it detoxifies; is diuretic and sudorific; stimulates bile secretion; is anticonvulsant, slightly soothing, a mild tonic, and helps wounds heal. Folk medicine prescribes it to treat headaches, liver problems, spleen conditions; to help with passing kidney or bladder stones; to strengthen the heart; and to improve sleep. It is also said to promote blood flow, inhibit inflammation, and strengthen the venous walls, thus helping venous conditions (Köbl 1993, 315). The wonderfully aromatic dry herb was also stuffed into the herbal pillow traditionally placed near mothers and babies during childbirth.

When I was a child in Germany in the early 1950s, it was typical to go for a family outing in the countryside on Sundays or holidays. If we stopped at an inn for a snack, my father would usually have a beer, my mother would have coffee, and the kids would order *Brause,* a fizzy soft drink. The choice was between a red, raspberry-flavored *Brause* or a green one flavored with woodruff. Cola and other soft drinks have since replaced these sodas, and the green woodruff soda was eventually banned on the grounds that it contains too much coumarin, which is said to contain carcinogens and be highly toxic for the liver. The renowned phytotherapist Dr. Rudolf Fritz Weiss, however, says it is not a health risk. He cites several animal experiments in which even after administration of coumarin active ingredients in tenfold and hundredfold doses, the malformation rate was not increased compared with the control group. He states: "According to this study, we can be completely reassured about the use of plants containing coumarin" (Weiss 2001, 253). Unfortunately, there is no real woodruff soda anymore. The Polish king Stanislaus Leszczynski (eighteenth century), an enlightened man and a patron of the arts, was once asked what the secret was to his long life and good health. He answered: woodruff tea; he drank a little cup of it every morning.

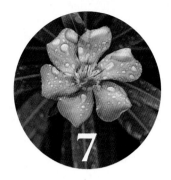

7

MODERN HEART PLANTS

The erroneous idea that plants and isolated active principles are equivalent has become a fixed dogma in pharmacology and medicine today.

ANDREW WEIL, *HEALING AND SELF-HEALING*

THERE ARE NOW MORE THAN A HUNDRED different types of cardiovascular or cardiotonic drugs that can help the cardiovascular system and the stressed heart that may be heading toward a heart attack. Particularly suitable plants are those with toxic glycosides that can split into a partial steroidal agglutinin (aglycone or adenosine, a nonsugar) and another part sugar (for example, rhamnose, digitoxose). In their molecular structure, the active substances resemble steroids and are like sex hormones, bile acids, cholesterol, and vitamin D (Schmidsberger 1990, 52). Correctly dosed, these heart glycosides strengthen and slow down the heartbeat—the heart races less. By increasing the stroke volume, they improve the blood circulation in the kidneys and increase urination. This also helps reduce venous congestion and fluid retention (edema).

Plants with cardiac glycosides are often found in the figwort family (Scrophulariaceae), such as foxglove;* the dogbane family (Apocynaceae),

---

*Since 2005, botanists classify the foxglove as a member of the plantain family (Plantaginaceae) and no longer as a member of the figwort family (Scrophulariaceae).

such as oleander (*Nerium oleander*), yellow oleander (*Thevetia peruviana*), and especially strophanthus; members of the buttercup family (Ranunculaceae), such as adonis and hellebore; and additionally, plants of the lily family (Liliaceae) are used, such as sea squill or lily of the valley. Based on the molecular structure of the cardiac glycosides, a distinction is made between the cardenolides (*Adonis, Convallaria, Digitalis, Nerium, Strophanthus, Thevetia*) with a five-membered lactone ring and the bufadienolides (*Helleborus, Urginea*) with a six-membered lactone ring. All these plants are highly toxic and as such hardly play a role in folk medicine.

In other plants effective for cardiovascular diseases, additional active substances, such as flavonoids, bitter substances, and alkaloids, are at work. These include, for example, Scotch broom (*Cytisus scoparius*), coffee, white hellebore (*Veratrum album*), periwinkle (*Vinca minor*), Indian snakeroot (*Rauvolfia serpentina*), and tobacco.

Rudolf Fritz Weiss divides medicinal plants into three categories:

1. *Mite* remedies: These are low-potency medicinal plants that act in the long term to regulate and prevent disease as well as being suitable for the treatment of chronic conditions and rehabilitation. They are safe to use because they are nontoxic and have few side effects. As for the active ingredients, these are mostly complex natural substance mixtures.
2. *Media* remedies: These are medications effective for acute conditions and may also be slightly toxic.
3. *Forte* remedies: These are used in medicine to achieve fast, powerful effects. What is effective in forte remedies are not complex molecular mixtures. Contrary to mite remedies, forte remedies are often powerful mono substances (alkaloids, glycosides). There is a risk of side effects with forte remedies.

The cardiac glycosides favored by conventional medicine belong, in the categorization of Rudolf Fritz Weiss, mainly to the forte remedies. He counts the lily of the valley (*Convallaria*) and the Adonis flower as media remedies. Heart-calming and preventive plants, such as lemon balm, valerian, lavender, ginkgo, motherwort, sloe, passionflower, garlic, mistletoe, onion, and hawthorn are among the mite remedies.

The heart, circulatory system, and blood vessels form a functional circuit; one cannot examine them in isolation. Therefore, even medicinal plants that do not act directly on the heart muscle can be regarded as modern heart plants. These include, for example, those that are suitable for borderline hypertension, such as garlic, mistletoe, snakeroot, onion, and hawthorn; and even those that can act on low blood pressure, such as ginseng, lavender, and rosemary. It also includes those that play a role in venous disorders, such as horse chestnut (*Aesculus hippocastanum*), butcher's broom (*Ruscus aculeatus*), and witch hazel (*Hamamelis virginiana*). Meadowsweet (*Filipendula ulmaria*), which improves the blood flow, and blood-thinning plants, such as sweet clover (*Meliolotus officinalis*), also deserve mention.

HEART PLANTS
WITH CARDIAC GLYCOSIDES

Attention! Laypersons and those who are inclined to self-medication are well advised to keep their hands off powerful plants such as the ones listed here. These contain poisons (cardiotoxins) that can lead to cardiac arrest at too high a dosage. The following are some of the most important plants native to northern Europe that have heart-effective glycosides and are only to be used by qualified professionals.

Foxglove
(*Digitalis purpurea*)

"Greetings, pale thimble,
I came to pick you,
that you restore my health,
because I have a goiter."

FOLK CHARM FROM LOWER BRITTANY
FOR COLLECTING FOXGLOVE

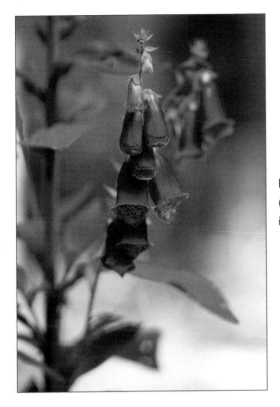

Foxglove
(*Digitalis purpurea*)
in full blossom

Who can deny the magic of the beautiful foxglove blooming at the edge of the forest at midsummer? An aura of enchantment surrounds this member of the figwort family (Scrophulariaceae). The common name in German, *Fingerhut* (thimble), suggests an elves' thimble; English common names include fairy thimbles, fairy bells, fairy cap, and fairy finger.* Above all, it is the purplish (rarely white), zygomorphous blossoms, with their deep brown-and-white-rimmed spots, that evoke the image of fairies and elves.† *Méaracáin na mBan Sí,* "Banshee's thimbles," is the name

---

*It has been suggested (cf. Davidson 1992, 267) that the name foxglove (Old English *foxes glófa*) may be a malapropism that evolved from the earlier *folces gleow,* with the first element, *folces,* "folk's," referring to the wee folk (nature spirits, fairies, and elves), and the second element, *gleow,* meaning "music, mirth, joy" (our modern word *glee* derives from this latter term). Over time, through a process of etymological reinterpretation, *folces* became "fox's" and *gleow* became "glove."

†Zygomorphous describes a part of a plant that has only one plane of symmetry—in other words, it is bilaterally symmetrical.

of the wildflower in Irish, and it is *lus nam ban-sith*, "herb of the fairy woman," in Scots Gaelic.

Foxglove is biennial. It blooms in the bright midsummer. Clusters of bell-shaped flowers always hang on the top of the stem and on the side of the strongest light incidence. Large bumblebees pollinate the blossoms. The heart-shaped seed capsules each contain several tens of thousands of tiny seeds (10,000 seeds weigh one gram). These seeds are light germinators. In its essence, the plant moves between light and shadow, lightness and heaviness. As a mediator of these polarities, it carries the signature of the heart, which also rhythmically beats between lightness and heaviness, flowing air, and flowing blood. When the heartbeat in the human microcosm weakens and threatens to fade, then the macrocosm offers this plant as an aid.

The unusually deep reddish-purple flowers of the foxglove are similar to the hollow organ of an animal. Usually, plants have no internal organs. As the German writer (and plant enthusiast) Johann Wolfgang von Goethe already observed, plant tissue is flat and directed toward the outside world. Foxglove is not only a living, growing being, but—as the flowers suggest—it is almost animated or "astralized." It is this animation that makes us stop and marvel at it when walking through the forest, and which evokes associations with fairies.

Foxglove thrives in the northwestern European-Atlantic climate.* Therefore, it was well known (and sacred) to the Celts but unknown in the Mediterranean. Neither the writings of classical antiquity nor those of monastic medicine mention foxglove. Celtic healers, such as the Welsh Meddygon Myddfai (twelfth century), used this fairy plant, mashed, externally as a poultice to eliminate tumors, pus, fever, and inflammation. Foxglove is still known in Germany as *Schwulstkraut* (tumor herb) and in Aveyron, Occitania (southern France), as *èrbo dé désènfladuro* (also meaning tumor herb). This is because the plant was

---

*The woolly foxglove (*Digitalis lanata*), favored today by the chemical-pharmaceutical industry because it can be cultivated in fields, is originally native to the steppe areas of the Black Sea and the Balkans.

used to heal tumors caused by snakebites. It was also referred to and used elsewhere as a "snake herb" (Marzell 1943–1979, II:135).

The botanist Leonhart Fuchs, who in 1542 was the first to name the plant *digitalis* ("thimble," based on Latin *digitus*, "finger"), had no knowledge about the cardiac efficacy of this forest plant. He wrote that the doctors of his time hardly know how to use it. He described its strengths and characteristics: "The digitalis herbs, boiled and drunk, break up the coarse moisture in the body, cleanse and purify, and take away obstructions of the liver and other internal organs" (Fuchs 1543). In addition, women can bring on "their time" (menstruation) with it; boiled in wine and drunk, it drives poison out of the body (certainly a very dangerous practice!); mixed with honey and applied, it dispels stains and impurities from the face and body. This "breaking up of coarse moisture" describes the plant as a purging and purifying agent, a remedy that purifies by producing vomiting, diarrhea, urinary urgency, and cold sweat. It has probably always been used in folk medicine as a purgative and antitumor agent.

Not until the time of the Industrial Revolution in the late eighteenth century did the English country doctor William Withering (1741–1799) discover the cardiac efficacy of foxglove. Withering was

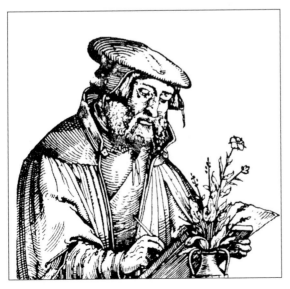

Leonhart Fuchs
(*De historia stirpium commentarii insignes*, Basel, 1542)

a follower of the then modern "heroic medicine," which rejected the herbalism of folk medicine as unscientific and practiced its craft with only mineral poisons (mercury, arsenic), purgatives, the scalpel, and bloodletting. Nevertheless, he had a soft spot for botany. His fiancée, like many a bourgeois lady of the time, painted watercolor flower motifs, and he helped her to find suitable plants. In 1775, when the couple went for summer retreats in Shropshire, he met a dropsical woman with grotesquely swollen arms, legs, and feet. She asked him for help, and he prescribed some placebos, but he thought to himself that the patient would not live much longer. However, when he visited the village again a few weeks later, to his surprise, he saw the patient completely happy and well again. He wondered how that was possible and inquired. He was told that there was an *auld hag* ("old hag," meaning an herbal practitioner) who had administered an herbal concoction. Because the good doctor found it beneath his dignity to ask himself, he had the herbalist secretly observed. He discovered that the brew consisted of more than twenty different herbs. He examined the mixture and became convinced that the foxglove it contained was the effective ingredient. Unfortunately, he did not think it necessary to name the other "useless" herbs—an example of the reductionism under which pharmacological science suffers to this day.

Now, he set out to study the effect of the poisonous plant on animals. He fed it to turkeys, who painfully vomited their intestinal contents and died miserably. He then experimented with destitute patients, whom he treated with foxglove for free (!) at a clinic in Birmingham. As a result of his research, in 1785 he published the classic *An Account of the Foxglove, and Some of Its Medical Uses: With Practical Remarks on Dropsy and Other Diseases* and thus became the "founder of cardiac therapy." Withering did not know that dropsy, the accumulation and congestion of fluid in the tissues, is not a disease in itself but the symptom of heart or kidney failure. Only later did it become clear that digitalis preparations corrected irregular heartbeat and cardiac contraction (systole). These preparations contain glycosides, which increase the pumping capacity of the heart, thereby accelerating the blood circulation and flushing out water congestion through increased urination (Pahlow 1979, 134). From the mid-nineteenth century onward, it increasingly became the medical fashion to "digitalize" patients with a weak heart. There were often failures. Digitalis poisoning became the most common iatrogenic cause of death at the time. Until 1914, foxglove was given in the form of dried leaf powder, and then standardized doses were synthetically produced—first digitoxin, then digoxin. For these toxic drugs, the safety factor is so tight that it is considered very important in medical school that students can accurately identify the symptoms of an overdose. They learn to pay attention to three consecutive stages of digitalis toxicity:

1st stage: gastrointestinal discomfort, nausea, and vomiting
2nd stage: arrhythmias in the atria of the heart
3rd stage: life-threatening ventricular arrhythmia, in which the heart chambers beat irregularly (Weil 1983, 103)

The well-known American physician Andrew Weil was surprised that he never saw the first stage of digoxin overdoses. First, there was no nausea or vomiting, just atrial arrhythmias that only became noticeable on the electrocardiogram. Later he realized that the first stage was only apparent when the herbal drug was administered. From then on, Dr. Weil treated cases of heart failure with the plant itself. If he over-administered, the patients first got an upset stomach. Then he was able to reduce the drug without the patients even coming close to arrhythmia. In this way, he could determine the individual dosage very accurately. Dr. Weil arrived at the following conclusion:

The whole plant has certain built-in safety mechanisms that are lost when the cardiotonic elements are refined out and used in pure form. Call this the wisdom of nature if you like, or don't if you don't like; it remains an empirical truth. (Weil 1983, 105)

Hellebore
(*Helleborus niger, H. viridis, H. foetidus*)

The English poet Robert Burton (1577–1640) wrote in his *Anatomie of Melancholy* (1621) concerning hellebore:

> *Borage* and *hellebor* fill two sceanes,
> Soveraigne plants to purge the veines
> Of melancholy, and cheare the heart,
> Of those blacke fumes which make it smart. (Burton
> 1628, frontispiece)

Chemists have now discovered that the rhizomes of the hellebore species contain the steroid saponin mixture helleborin and several alkaloids. Green hellebore, in particular, contains hellebrin, a bufadienolide (toad poison), which in its cardiac efficacy corresponds to the strophantus glycosides (Ammon 2004, 711). Thus, the green hellebore would be a modern heart plant. However, because the glycoside content of the highly toxic plant varies greatly and the effect is less controllable, it is no longer used in conventional medicine, except in homeopathic preparation.

The Christmas rose (*Helleborus niger*), growing wild in the eastern limestone Alps, is known primarily as a garden plant. The hellebore, which we encounter in the Jura Mountains and on limestone soils north of the Alps, is either the stinking hellebore (*H. foetidus*) or the green hellebore (*H. viridis*). In the past, however, there was little differentiation among the different types of hellebores, and they were all used in the same way.

The hellebore species live contrary to the rest of nature. In late autumn, when the trees drop their foliage, and most other flowers wither and seeds form, the hellebore begins to develop flower buds. Finally, at the winter solstice, when the sun reaches its low point, they open their flowers—that is why the white-flowered *Helleborus niger* is also called the Christmas rose. With pink-tinged, greenish-white petals

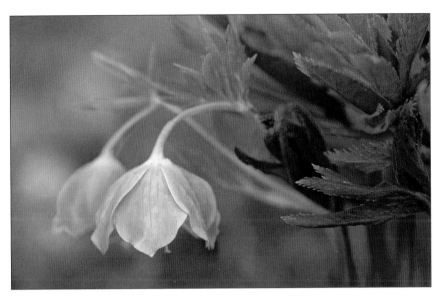

Green hellebore (*H. viridis*) leaves and early blossoms

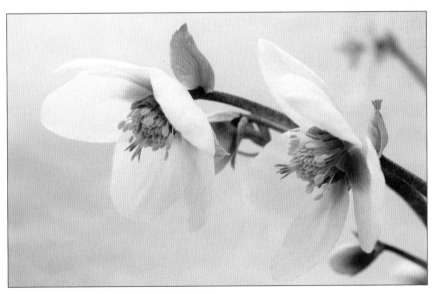

Black hellebore (*H. niger*), or Christmas rose, blossoms

and honey scent, it lures the last insects before they freeze. And if the insects happen to stay away, the plant pollinates itself.

Does nature present a sign with this "snow-rose" that despite the sad and saturnine cold season, the reincarnation of light will mysteriously take place? Does it wish to welcome the Christ Child—who appears in the dead of night as a sort of inner sun—with its blossoms? A poet or mystic might interpret it so.

Like the autumn crocus (or meadow saffron) or the ivy, which continues to bloom on into the winter, the hellebore is a poisonous plant. It is often the case that plants that rebel against the natural rhythm of the sun are highly toxic. In fact, the hellebore contains various poisons: black hellebore has protoanemonin, which irritates the kidneys and mucous membranes; contact with the fresh, wounded plant can cause disruptions in the nervous system similar to the effects of a ganglionic blocker. The green and stinking hellebore varieties contain even more of the cardiac glycoside hellebrin, which—like digitalis—affects the rhythm and power of the heart, the "microcosmic sun." In addition, there are saponins, which have a strongly irritating effect on the mucous membranes, cause nausea, and have drastically laxative effects. The toxic reaction is awful. It ranges from excessive salivation, nausea, and vomiting to severe stomach and intestinal pain, diarrhea, dizziness, tinnitus, blindness, twitching, labored breathing, and a weak pulse. The poisoning finally ends in convulsions or even death. But it is just this poisonous effect, this eerie power of the root in particular, that makes the hellebore one of the most important medicinal plants. Whether a plant is a remedy or poison is—as Paracelsus taught—primarily a matter of dosage.

Together with other poisons, such as monkshood, the black hellebore root was mixed into bait for wolves and foxes. But above all, it was regarded as a valuable means of purification. Emetics, laxatives, and sudorifics represent some of the oldest and most universal therapies. The root was probably already used in the Stone Age. The Greeks were known to ingest the root powder in honey mead or cedar oil to divert "bad fluids," snake venom, and worms out of the body.

The dried root powder was also snorted: the ensuing explosive sneeze forced out the demonic, malignant entities that had been housing themselves deeply in the body (even in the bones and marrow, it was believed). It was given to those who were possessed, insane, and epileptic. It was even sprinkled into chimneys—traditionally known to be an entrance route for spirits—to keep unpleasant otherworldly entities out of the home.

The ecstatic-orgiastic cult of Dionysus, which originated in Asia and swept over Greece some 2,500 years ago, caused great concern to the patriarchs of the city-states. The wine god, decorated with ivy and snakes, brought more and more people—especially young women—under his spell. Possessed by the wine demon and contemptuous of all good manners, they meandered through the woods, drunk and rampant, celebrating wild and often bloody orgies. Melampus of Pylos, a seer and priest of the sun god Apollo, was charged with controlling the excesses of the wine demon. He gave the ecstatic daughters of the patricians the milk of goats who had eaten hellebore leaves. The girls became sober at once. Since then, the pungent plant of the buttercup family (Ranunculaceae) has also been called the Melampode.

Of course, such a powerful root should not be carelessly dug out of the ground. It requires an elaborate ritual so that the plant spirit, which can appear in the form of an eagle, is not displeased. Whoever wants to dig the root first draws a circle around the plant. Turning his head to the east, he prays to Apollo and then to Asclepius, the Great Healer. He should eat some garlic, drink a glass of unsweetened wine, and then dig quickly, because the smell of the root causes one to become heavy-headed.

The physicians of antiquity, from Hippocrates to Dioscorides, followed the ancient magical folk tradition when they prescribed hellebore to their patients to induce beneficial vomiting, purging, and urination. The theoretical framework of their humoralism was the four-fluids doctrine. According to this theory, the human body consists of four cardinal fluids, or "humors," which in turn are connected to the elements, the seasons, the patient's age, a major organ, and the temperament.

CORRESPONDENCES OF THE FOUR HUMORS

	RED BLOOD	YELLOW BILE	WHITE MUCUS	BLACK BILE
Quality	Sweet, warm, moist	Warm, bitter, dry	Salty, cold, moist	Pungent, cold, dry
Element	Air	Fire	Water	Earth
Season	Spring	Summer	Fall	Winter
Age	Childhood	Adolescence	Maturity	Old age
Organ	Heart	Liver	Brain	Spleen
Temperament	Sanguine	Choleric	Phlegmatic	Melancholic

When all the humors are in balance, then a person is healthy—he or she has "good humor." However, if some fluids dominate, these must be eliminated, routed, or purged. In this case, a plant like hellebore can be a true godsend. As a sneezing powder it pulls the mucus out, as an emetic, the yellow bile. For females, hellebore promotes the monthly menstruation and may even cause an abortion. Above all, it purges black bile, which has its proper seat in the digestive system but can darken the heart and even rise to the brain. According to the principle "like attracts like," the black, corrosive root attracts this harmful fluid and passes it via the spleen into the intestine, where it is quickly excreted.

These doctors of old endeavored to understand diseases and remedies in a cosmic context. Any suffering caused by the unfavorable influence of a planet was treated with a medicinal herb that also bears the signature of the planet. In the case of hellebore, it was clear: it belongs to Saturn, the slowest of the visible planets, the old man among them. In nature, it manifests in the dark, gray, cold year's end—the time when this plant blooms. Saturn governs old age: in the positive aspect as wisdom, sobriety, and serenity; in the negative aspect as melancholy, old age, calcification, and severe infirmity. The Greek physician Dioscorides, who authored the first European herbal in the first century CE, used hellebore for traumatic conditions such

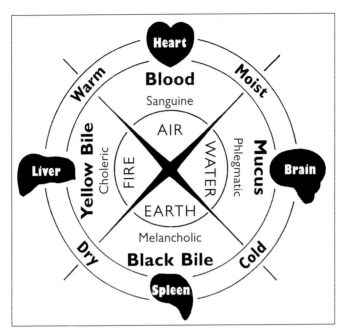

The four humors (after R. Herrlinger, 1961)

as gout, deafness, chronic constipation, and scabies. "The miser first: none wants a keeper more / Or asks a stronger dose of hellebore," wrote Horace (*Satires* II, 3)—and what trait of the soul could be more saturnine than miserliness?

Of course, the Saturn plant should be dug up on Saturn's day (Saturday), at Saturn's hour—that is, at a time when the planet is in its own house or otherwise well aspected.

Because of its toxicity, hellebore gradually came into disrepute. Worming and delousing cures, abortions, and treatments of the possessed or the epileptic were often fatal. Also, black hellebore (*Helleborus niger*) was often enough confused with the so-called white hellebore, (*Veratrum album,* false helloborine). However, black hellebore did continue to be used in veterinary medicine to treat red murrain. The farmers bored a hole in the sick pig's ear and stuck in a piece of the root.

At the beginning of the modern era, Paracelsus rediscovered the plant. Full of enthusiasm, he wrote in his *Herbarius*: "There is more virtue and power in this herb than any of the writers, who are read in higher schools, have ever written regarding longevity." According to Paracelsus, a doctor who alone knows how to use this plant properly has sufficient knowledge. The hellebore "removes from the body what is not supposed to be in it" (Pörksen 1988, 27). The root has the power to drive off four diseases: epilepsy, gout, stroke, and dropsy. Above all, Paracelsus saw in the leaves an "elixir of long life." This is what the old philosophers did: dried the leaves in the east wind, then ground them to powder with an equal amount of fine sugar. One should take a quarter of a lot (2.1 grams) every morning until the sixtieth to the seventieth year of life; between the seventieth and eightieth year, the same amount every two days; and after the age of eighty, every sixth day. (Beware! That is a high dose!)

Also, in German folk medicine it is said: "Anyone who carries a piece of the Christmas rose root on his person will live to a very old age." So maybe there's something to that old recipe? Dr. Rudolf Fritz Weiss, the modern founder of phytotherapy, wrote that this is certainly the case; it concerns the administration of a cardiac glycoside in *very small quantities*: "Paracelsus had obviously very correctly discovered that the dried leaves were better tolerated than preparations made from the roots" (Weiss 2001, 244).

Lily of the Valley
(*Convallaria majalis*)

"With the dew of the May bells,
the maiden washes her face,
bathes her golden locks."

LUDWIG UHLAND

In April and May, the lovely, sweetly scented, snow-white and bell-shaped blossoms of the lily of the valley, also known as may bells, open. The flowers—which grow wild in open deciduous woodlands in the cool northern climates of Europe and Asia, thermophilic pine forests, mountain meadows, and in underbrush—are a sure sign of the relief from win-

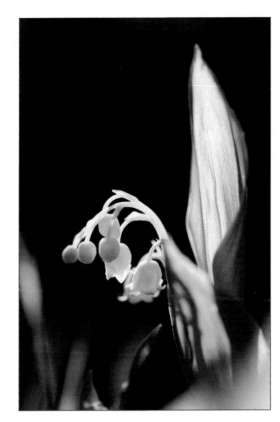

Lily of the valley
(*Convallaria majalis*)
leaves and blossoms

ter cold and cloudiness. *Convallaria majalis* var. *montana* grows wild in North America. Not much has been written about it, but certainly the delicate lily plant once played a role in folk customs and religion. It was probably dedicated to the goddesses of spring—the Germanic Ostara; the Celtic Olwen, whose name means "white trail"; or the Slavic Marena—who drive the winter away. In any case, it belonged to the May festival, the wedding celebration of the radiant sun god (Belenos) and his flower-decorated May bride, the goddess of the plants. In Paris, May 1st is still the "lily-of-the-valley day" (*la journée du muguet*), and whoever wears the flower on that day will be lucky all year round.

It did not take the Christians long to adopt the pure white flower as an attribute of the gentleness and purity of the Virgin Mary. Mary's tears and Our Lady's tears are other names of the plant, for it is said to have sprung from the tears that Mother Mary shed under the cross of her son. Medieval monks christened the plant *lilium convallium,* "lily of the valley," remembering the Song of Solomon (2:1–3): "I am the rose of Sharon / And the lily of the valleys. / Like a lily among thorns, / So is my love among the daughters." On medieval panel paintings, lilies of the valley also appear as attributes of the Son of Mary: the pure white flowers symbolize his purity and innocence; the scarlet berries ripening in the autumn represent his redeeming blood.

The lily of the valley seems to have been unknown to the physicians of antiquity; it is not mentioned in ancient texts. Only in the sixteenth century did the plant appear in herbals. Hieronymus Brunschwig mentions in his "Distillery Book" (*Liber de arte distillandi, de simplicibus*) that "May-bell water" was good against poison and fainting; strengthens the heart, senses, and brain; stops the shakes when rubbed on the hands and arms; a tea helps with incontinence and can cure an inflamed liver; and so on (Madaus 1979, 1091). Soon thereafter the lily of the valley became a veritable modern therapy of the times; it was considered extremely effective and was referred to as *salus mundi,* "salvation of the world." Doctors even took the flower as the emblem of their profession; they were portrayed with the lily of the valley or decorated their coats-of-arms with the white bell-blossoms. Copernicus, who had studied medicine in Padua, is depicted on a woodcut with a lily of the valley in his hand. The inscription reads:

> *Copernicus als Artz ziert ihn ein Mayen-Strauß;*
> *Er rechnete der Welten Laufbahn aus . . .*

> Copernicus as doctor, a May-bouquet decorated;
> He worked out the orbit of the planets . . .

According to the teachings of the time, the lily of the valley contains a volatile salt that is mercurial and even has sulfurous constituents, which strengthen the spirit, but especially the brain, the nerves, and the nerve fluid. Consequently, it was an excellent remedy for all head diseases such as dizziness, severe distress (epilepsy), somnolence, melancholy, and apoplexy.* Sneezing powder was prepared from the flowers to cleanse the brain. Folk medicine also used the lily of the valley to treat headaches, dizziness, dropsy, and stroke; to treat rabies, a decoction of the plant was drunk and applied as a poultice. Inflamed eyes were flushed with a lily of the valley concoction, and one could supposedly make freckles disappear with the flowers picked before dawn. In Russian folk medicine, the flowers were macerated in brandy for three months and given in drops to cure epilepsy (Madaus 1979, 1092). The roots, which have warming and dispersing power, could break up and dispel "all clotted and stagnant blood, resulting from contusions, falling accidents, blows, and similar mishaps," as well as birthmarks and stains, and furthermore generate delicate, white skin (Hovorka and Kronfeld 1909, 284). Root preparations were also used against leukorrhea and impotence. The folklorists Oskar von Hovorka and Adolf Kronfeld, in their account of the traditional applications of the lily of the valley, commented: "Oddly enough, we find very little mention of the influence of the plant on the heart's activity, and only the general statement that the distillates are used to strengthen the heart. The plant is indeed a cardiac remedy of scientific medicine" (Hovorka and Kronfeld 1909, 284).

The medical Convallaria fad ebbed in the seventeenth century, and by the eighteenth century lily of the valley had completely disappeared from the drug arsenal. It was not until the end of the nineteenth century that the drug was reexamined, particularly in Russia, and the efficacy of the flower tincture in cardiac neuroses and seizure-related symptoms of cardiac angina was recognized (Madaus 1979, 1093). The French physician G. Sée introduced the diuretic drug into his practice and had success with several different heart conditions. He used it primarily as a cardiac sedative for nervous conditions.

Meanwhile, we know that lily of the valley strengthens the heartbeat while at the same time slowing down and regulating the rhythm. Convallaria contains about forty glycosides (cardenolides), including

---

*Apoplexy refers to sudden paralysis or stroke; according to the humoral theory, during apoplexy a "drop" falls into the brain.

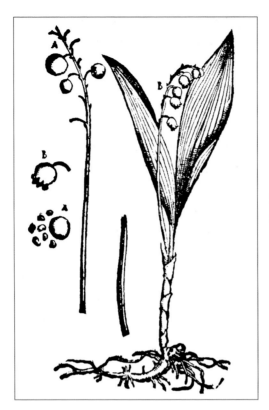

Lily of the valley
(*Convallaria majalis*)

the pure glycoside convallatoxin, and eight different flavonoids, which do not give the best results as pure substances but only in their interaction. The flavonoids in lily of the valley expand the blood vessels, and the asparagine acts diuretically. The cardiac glycoside convallatoxin can compete with strophanthin; it works quickly, but it decomposes quickly and is well excreted by the kidneys so that no toxic accumulation occurs (Weiss 2001, 199). Arrhythmia is not to be feared. According to Rudolf Fritz Weiss, the drug may be considered for mild and moderate forms of heart failure; however, it cannot replace digitalis in cases of severe insufficiency.* Lily of the valley is especially

---

*Dr. Rudolf Fritz Weiss (1885–1991) worked tirelessly to bring herbal medicine back into medical practice. His German textbook of phytotherapy, published in English as *Weiss's Herbal Medicine* (New York: Thieme, 2001), is considered a classic of the literature.

good for tachycardic forms of heart failure (Weiss and Fintelmann 2002, 167). Extracts of Convallaria support hawthorn treatment in the case of an aging heart.

Gerhard Madaus wrote:

> Convallaria is a good cardiac remedy that resembles digitalis in its effect. It differs from digitalis in that it has lower adhesion to the heart muscle and a greater vascular effect. . . . With edema and severe congestion, digitalis will always be preferred. On the other hand, the nervous heart complaints . . . can be better treated with Convallaria than with digitalis. (Madaus 1979, 1097)

Because all parts of lily of the valley are poisonous, irritating the digestive tract and causing nausea and vomiting, the layperson should leave the application to the trained herbalist or doctor. However, anyone can wear the fragrant flowers on their hat to let the world know that they have rediscovered happiness in love.

Oleander
(*Nerium oleander*)

Oleander, a well-known and beautiful plant of the dogbane family, is a native of the Mediterranean but can be found worldwide as a non-indigenous plant in subtropical regions. Because of its white, pink, or reddish-purple flowers, it can be seen around the world as a potted ornamental. With its lovely scent that smells like vanilla or jasmine, in the evenings it attracts moths with a long proboscis. However, this small tree, which blossoms and smells so beautifully, is a highly poisonous plant. For this reason, it was once considered a symbol of falsehood. The Greeks believed that oleander came from the magical garden of the poisoner Medea of Colchis. It is known that Alexander the Great had recurring problems with oleander on his campaigns because the pack animals, donkeys, and horses who had gnawed on it would die. Gustav Hegi reported about twelve French soldiers who roasted their

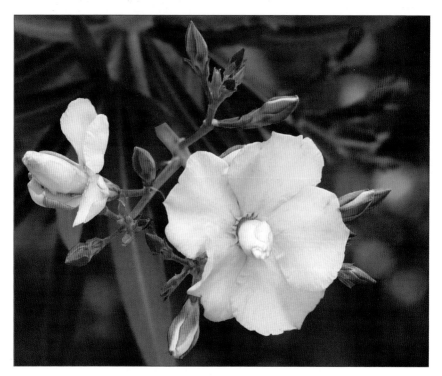

Oleander (*Nerium oleander*) blossoms

meat rations on oleander spears in Spain in 1808—eight died, and four became seriously ill (Hegi 1906–1931, V / 3:2057). The plant is so poisonous that mice die from simply biting through the leaves. In Greece, oleander leaves are still stuffed into the holes of the undesirable rodents. It was believed, however, that such a poisonous plant, when cooked in wine—following the principle of "like cures like" (*similia similibus curentur*)—acts as an antidote for snakebites.

In Mediterranean and Arabian folk medicine, a decoction of oleander leaves is used externally to eliminate skin parasites and scabies, and tinctures are taken internally to abort unwanted children. The cardiac efficacy of oleander is based on digitalis-like cardenolide glycosides. Their effect was first discovered in 1866 by the Russian researcher M. E. Pelikan. The leaves, harvested before the bush has blossomed, were formerly used to treat heart failure and functional heart disorders. Nerium received a negative monograph from

Commission E; consequently its medical use has been prohibited in some European countries.*

Queen of the Night
(*Selenicereus grandiflorus*)

Also known as night blooming cereus, this slender, five- to six-sided cactus, which is a popular houseplant, comes from the semi-deserts of the Caribbean and Central America. The plant was named after Selene, the Greek moon goddess, and Cereus, which means "wax" or "wax torch." It opens its large, vanilla-scented, yellow-pollen-filled flower crown with ivory-white petals only once a year for just one night. For those who experience this flowering miracle, it has an almost erotic component. Allegedly, the flowers, when taken by women, have an aphrodisiac effect and they, too, will blossom that night for their lover just like this magical flower.

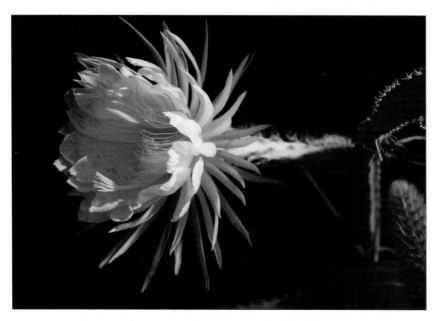

Queen of the night (*Selenicereus grandiflorus*) bloom

---

*See footnote on page 169.

Central American indigenous healers used this herb as a remedy for inflammation of the bladder and dropsy and the fresh juice externally as a helpful skin stimulant for rheumatic complaints (Hiller and Melzig 2003, 273). It was not until 1864 that the Italian physician Rubini discovered and publicized the cardiac efficacy of the cactus. Selenicereus is said to stimulate the contraction strength of the heart and expand the heart vessels and the peripheral vessels. Indications include indeterminate nervous heart complaints, angina pectoris, cardiac arrhythmia, and myocardial insufficiency. Flavonol glycosides and amines are said to be responsible for the effect. The queen of the night should not be taken directly as a tea but instead as a whole extract in ready-to-use preparations.

Spring Pheasant's Eye
(*Adonis vernalis*)

The spring pheasant's eye (*Adonis vernalis*), of the buttercup family (Ranunculaceae), stands under official plant protection. In the wild, it is found mainly in southeastern Europe and southern Russia on warm, dry limestone soils. Its bright, golden-yellow, sunlike flowers have been considered heralds of spring since antiquity. They were once dedicated to Adonis (from Phoenician *adon,* "lord"), a spring hero of antiquity and the lover of Aphrodite. After this young hunter was gored by a boar during a hunting trip—jealous Ares had sent the animal—he bled to death in the arms of the goddess. Where her tears mingled with his blood, the spring pheasant's eye appeared. In the Middle East of antiquity, the resurrection of the spring god was celebrated each year during a spring festival called the Adonia.

In Russian folk medicine, summer pheasant's eye (*A. aestivalis*) plays an important role. The dried, pulverized roots have been used traditionally as an emetic; the dried herb is used as a tea or decoction for dropsy, stone ailments, menstrual cramps, and febrile convulsion in infants. But it was not until the end of the nineteenth century that the Russian doctor and medical researcher A. N. Bubnov concluded that the plant

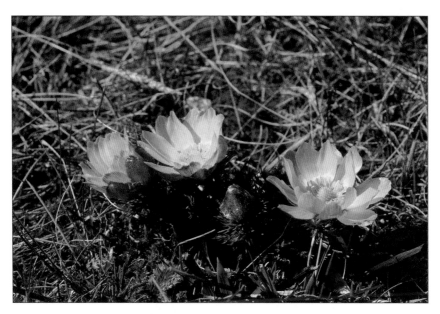

Spring pheasant's eye (*Adonis vernalis*) blossoms

only helps with dropsy if caused by a compensatory disturbance of heart activity. He noted that spring pheasant's eye has a digitalis-like effect, but no cumulative side effects, and that its therapeutic effect does not weaken, even with prolonged use (Madaus 1979, 408). The cardioactive glycosides (cardenolides) strengthen the contractility of the heart. But there is also a centrally sedating component that calms a nervous, racing heart. In addition, spring pheasant's eye expands the coronary vessels and tonifies the veins. Overdose causes nausea, vomiting, and cardiac arrhythmias.

Squill
(*Scilla maritima, Urginea maritima*)

White squill, a hyacinth plant, is native to the shores of the Mediterranean Sea. Red squill is common in Algeria and Morocco. Squill is also known as sea onion.

White squill is a perennial with white blossoms that are arranged grape-like around the stem and a fist-size, scaly onion bulb. It contains

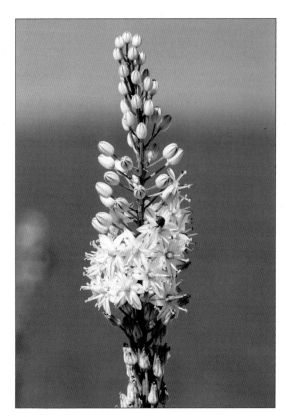

White squill, the sea onion (*Scilla maritima, Urginea maritima*)

about fifteen cardioactive glycosides that are classified as toad-venom-related bufadienolides, some of which are also found in the hellebore. The ingredients in white squill are particularly suitable for people with heart disease who cannot tolerate cardenolides (digitalis, convallaria, Adonis, nerium). As a medicament, scilla strengthens cardiac output and has a strong diuretic effect; it is suitable for the treatment of heart failure with concomitant renal insufficiency. For rodents, these glycosides are a strong neurotoxin. The red variety produces a highly effective rat poison.

Squill was already used in ancient Egypt, as we learn from the Ebers Papyrus (ca. 1500 BCE). Pliny and Dioscorides recommended it for dropsy. The humoral pathologists used the drug, which is considered warm and dry, to clear out mucus and to treat asthma, coughing, constipation, swelling of the spleen, malaria, and jaundice.

Wallflower
(*Erysimum cheiri*)

The wallflower, a relative of cabbage (Brassicaceae family), is originally at home in southern Europe. Because of its strongly fragrant and beautiful yellow, orange, or reddish-brown flowers, it is a popular garden plant. It also grows wild in warmer regions on limestone soils, where viticulture also thrives.

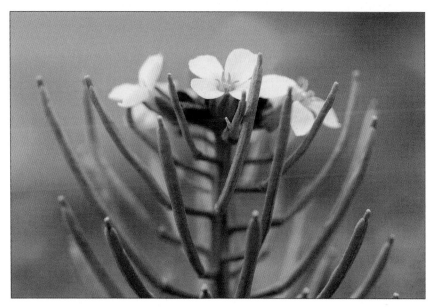

Wallflower (*Erysimum cheiri*) blossoms and immature seed capsules

The physicians of antiquity, such as Hippocrates and Dioscorides, knew the wallflower mainly as a remedy for female disorders. They prescribed the dried and then boiled flowers as a sitz bath, or hip bath, to treat inflammation of the uterus; and the seeds, taken internally to promote menstruation, induce abortion, or to expel the afterbirth. Even the herbalists of the Middle Ages used them in this way. Paracelsus used the wallflower to treat paralysis and consumption (Madaus 1979, 914). In folk medicine it was also used for liver disease, dropsy, and as a purgative and emmenagogue. As a medicament, the wallflower—especially

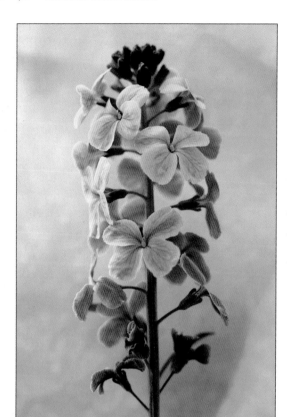

Wallflower in
full bloom

the seeds and flowers—contains cardioactive cardenolide glycosides
with a digitalis-like effect.

HEART PLANTS WITH ALKALOIDS
AND OTHER ACTIVE COMPONENTS

Garlic
(*Allium sativum*)

The garlic discussed previously was bear leek, also known as bear's garlic. But it should be mentioned again that garden garlic also reduces blood pressure, improves blood levels, prevents arteriosclerosis, reduces the risk of thrombosis, and promotes blood circulation.

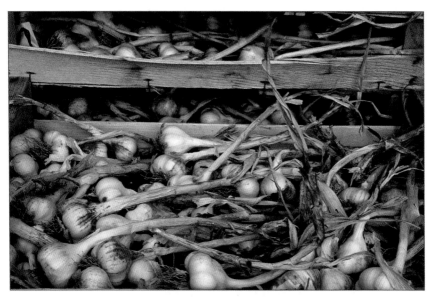

Harvested garlic bulbs drying in the sun

Hawthorn
(*Crataegus* spp.)

In 1850, a few decades after William Withering happened to discover the cardiac efficacy of foxglove, the Irish homoeopath Thomas Green conducted self-tests with hawthorn. He discovered a remedy for heart patients—the numbers of which were increasing in the wake of industrialization. His practice in Dublin became an insider tip for cardiac patients. How did Dr. Green come to this shrub or small tree? Perhaps it was his openness to the morphogenetic field of Ireland, the land of his ancestors, that led him to this discovery. Hawthorn hedgerows traverse the Emerald Isle and separate the pastures. For many centuries, as elsewhere in Europe, the hard, solid hawthorn wood has been turned, planed, and drilled to make hammers, ax handles, threshing flails, wooden gears (such as little drive wheels for mills), combs, walking sticks, and briar pipe bowls. The mealy red fruit was baked into bread as a flour additive, added to the pigs' feed, and brewed for a beer-like drink or even distilled into brandy; the root and bark served clothiers for dyeing textiles yellow.

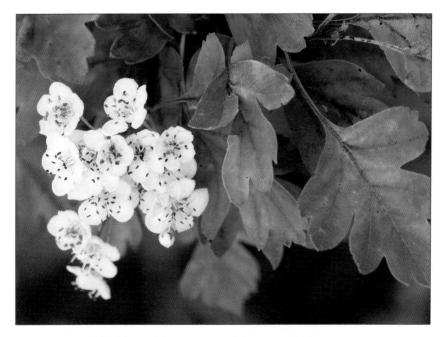

Hawthorn (*Crataegus* spp.) leaves and blossoms

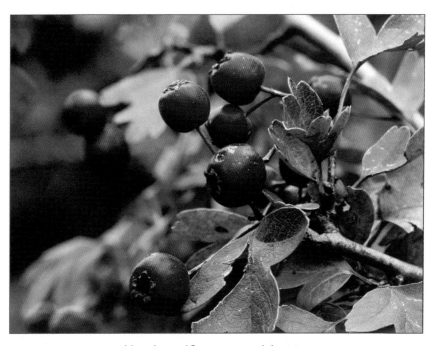

Hawthorn (*Crataegus* spp.) berries

But apart from these practical uses, hawthorn has always been considered a holy tree by the Irish and other Celtic peoples. It was one of the three "chieftain trees," the sacred trio—oak, ash, and hawthorn—and those who cut them down wantonly were severely punished. For the May Festival (Beltaine), the May Queen—one of the village's most beautiful maidens, who embodied the flower and sun goddess Olwen (the "golden wheel")—wore a splendid wreath of blossoming hawthorn. This orgiastic feast, celebrating the marriage of the goddess of vegetation to the sun god, took place when the full moon's light fell onto the blossoming hawthorn. The young woman was given to the strongest young lad—he personified Belenos, the sun hero—as a companion, and all were convinced that her presence would bless the fields abundantly with grain and the gardens with fruit (Storl 2000, 188).

In a Breton story, we learn that Merlin, the archetype of the Celtic druid, dreamed sweet dreams until the end of time while sleeping under an old hawthorn bush. The magician had fallen in love with the beautiful fairy Viviane (Nimue). She gently took the old wise man by the hand, wrapped him in her graceful arms like the ivy enwraps oak trees, and with sweet words elicited all his magical secrets from him. One day, lying down in the sacred grove of Belenos (Broceliande in Brittany) under the hawthorn, she asked him if he would tell her how a woman captivates a man without walls, towers, or chains, through the power of the spell alone, so that he could never escape her again. He told her. And when he had fallen asleep with his head in her lap, she accomplished the enchantment, just as he had taught her. Nine times she circled him; she repeated the magical words nine times. And since then, he sits, smiling like the Buddha, under the hawthorn. However, it would be wrong to believe that the enchanted one is unhappy. Among the branches of the hawthorn tree, the wise man of the forest found the female half of his being, the center of his heart.

For the Germanic peoples, the hawthorn hedge meant security. Protectively, it surrounds the farm and fields, providing safe sleep and good dreams. The hawthorn hedge was also the place where the old women gathered herbs and nine kinds of wood. In the early Middle

Ages, the *hagazussa* was to be found in the *hag* or hedge.* The Slavs recognized in the hawthorn a protection against bloodsucking vampires. They pierced the heart of a vampire's corpse, or any corpse feared to become one, with hawthorn stakes.

Although there are many folk customs and much folklore that surround this thorny bush, it did not play a major role in folk medicine. A mash of the berries may have been consumed for gastrointestinal influenza or diarrhea, and the hard seeds were crushed, boiled, and eaten to eliminate bladder and kidney stones. (The latter treatment was probably based on a misunderstanding of the plant's signature.) Otherwise, hawthorn twigs were laid on thresholds to keep witches away, and bewitched milk was beaten with hawthorn sticks to ward off the envy-driven magic that caused the problem.

Meanwhile, hawthorn is one of our best and easiest-to-tolerate nontoxic cardiovascular healing plants. The tea (infusion), or a ready-made preparation of flowers and leaves, is a wonderful remedy for nervous heart complaints, palpitations, extrasystole, sharp chest pains, and tightness in the chest. The scope of application includes aging heart, fatty heart, heart failure, hypertension, circulatory disorders, angina pectoris, and other forms of coronary heart disease. Above all, hawthorn stimulates the coronary blood flow. The impulse transfer from ganglion in the heart to the heart muscle cells is improved. The arterial vascular resistance in the heart as well as in the body is improved. The contraction force of the heart muscles is strengthened. This "mite-plant remedy" (according to Rudolf Fritz Weiss; see page 215) can be drunk for an extended period of time, over years: the two known side effects are protection against articular cartilage damage and improvement in arteriosclerosis. The fruits—which can also be added to the leaves for tea—improve the symptoms of chronic inflammatory bowel disease (Kaden 2007, 44). These effects

---

*The Old High German word *hagazussa* would eventually develop into the modern German word *Hexe*, "witch." The older term had a direct parallel in Old English *hægtesse*, likewise designating a "witch"; the first element of both words corresponds to "hag," which referred to the "haw" or hedge, while the second element referred to a witch or demon. The English word *hag* also took on the connotations of a witch.

are ascribed to the bioflavonoids rutin and quercetin. These increase the tone of the small blood vessels, diminish their permeability, and relax the arteries; they help regulate blood pressure and heartbeat and act as antioxidants. Other active ingredients include triterpenoids, procyanidins, the circulation-stimulating trimethylamine in the flowers, phenols, coumarins, and tannins.

There are apparently between 200 and 1,000 species and subspecies of hawthorn, which are sometimes difficult to distinguish from one another. They mainly grow in the temperate regions of the Northern Hemisphere. In Europe, there is especially the one-seed hawthorn (*Crataegus monogyna*), with a stylus and lobed leaves, and the two-eyed hawthorn (*Crataegus oxyacanthus*, syn. *C. laevigata*), which may also appear in a red-flowering variety as red hawthorn. Bastardized intermediate forms (hybrids) exist as well. For the herbalist, these differences are irrelevant; both are equally effective. Also, the various North American *Crataegus* species (*C. arnoldiana, C. diffusa, C. flava, C. mollis, C. prunifolia, C. phaenopyrum, C. punctata, C. viridis,* etc.), which often have longer, more robust thorns and larger fruit and grow partly as horticultural varieties, are all well suited as a heart remedy (Erichsen-Brown 1979, 155). The Native Americans especially collected the dried berries for their winter food supplies or used them—like the Chinese *Crataegus pinnatifida* (Chinese *Shan Zha*)—as a gastrointestinal remedy.

The hawthorn is a member of the rose family (Rosaceae) from the Crataegae tribe, which also includes cotoneaster, firethorn (pyracantha), and medlar. The small tree can live for about six hundred years; seed germination takes eighteen months. The hawthorn—also called quickthorn, May-tree, whitethorn, and hawberry—has, like many other rose plants, a generally strengthening, harmonizing, and tonic effect.

Mistletoe
(*Viscum album*)

The mistletoe, the magical plant of old that grows all over the world in various species, did not reveal its heart-effective qualities until recently.

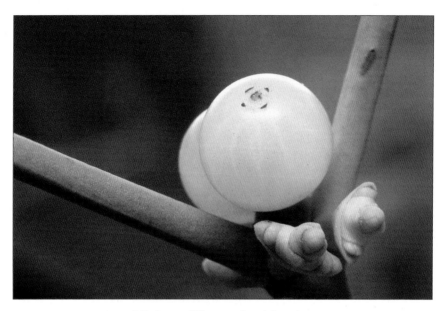

Mistletoe (*Viscum album*) berries

It was the French physician Gaulthier who discovered (in 1907) the antihypertensive effects of mistletoe extractions. The active ingredient is an acetylcholine-like choline derivative, which stimulates the parasympathetic nervous system, reducing blood pressure by subsequent vascular relief (Madaus 1979, 2838). Mistletoe tea, or a cold-water extract, or mistletoe drops are among the most popular remedies for treating hardening of the arteries and hypertension, as well as dizziness and tinnitus resulting from high blood pressure. Some authors speak of a harmonizing, adaptogenic effect: mistletoe lowers high blood pressure and raises low blood pressure. Rudolf Fritz Weiss mentions a tried-and-true "blood pressure tea" consisting of a mixture of mistletoe (to lower blood pressure), hawthorn (to promote coronary blood flow), and lemon balm (to calm the nervous heart) (Weiss and Fintelmann 2002, 191). It is probably because of this antihypertensive effect that the mistletoe was used by the Romans to help with epilepsy. The plant that grows high up on the trees was believed to help even with dizziness, epilepsy (earlier known as St. Valentine's disease), and St. Vitus's dance (Huntington's disease), which were fairly common in the Middle Ages.

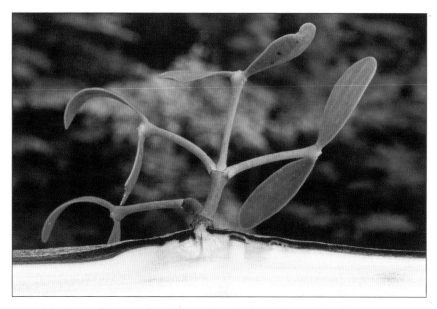

Mistletoe (*Viscum album*) branch with "roots" in bark of host tree

When powerful otherworldly beings approach the human soul, people can easily lose their minds, become dizzy, and the soul might even wander out of its bodily frame. In antiquity, physicians believed that the soul is catapulted out of the body during an epileptic seizure. In this case, magical medicine is needed. Mistletoe is one of these kinds of medicine because it is not a normal plant in terms of its appearance and habitus: the strange, parasitic showy mistletoe (Loranthaceae family) has emancipated itself from the normal cosmic-solar rhythm. It remains green despite winter cold, blooms while there is snow, and forms its fruits in November and December. The mistletoe cannot grow on the ground but only in the branches of trees. It has no real roots, but green "bark roots" that penetrate the tree bark, taking water and nutrients from it. It does not grow toward the sun, but forms an evergreen sphere, with the leaves never developing beyond the stage of the cotyledon. It cannot self-seed and relies on thrushes that transfer its sticky, slimy, poisonous berries to other trees. It has no bark, does not wither, and cannot heal its wounds.

It is neither tree nor herb. It is, as the Celts described it, something "in-between"—a being between this world and the otherworld, between heaven and earth. In the countries where Celtic culture has persisted for a longer time, the custom of hanging a mistletoe above the door frame (a liminal location between inside and outside) during the time of the winter solstice (the magical twelve days of Christmas, which liminally span between the old and the new year) is still kept up, even today. Anyone who happens to stand under the mistletoe is briefly freed from the rules of social behavior, and if two people meet there at the same time, a kiss is due. In such magical neither/nor spaces meaningful change, metamorphosis, or healing is possible.

As the Greek legend of Aeneas—who descended into the underworld with this "golden bough"—suggests, mistletoe also mediates between the realm of the living and the dead. The Scandinavian legend of Baldur also implies this. Baldur, the immortal sun god, can only be killed by mistletoe. The *hlaut-teinn* (lot-twig), the sacrificial frond or twig of mistletoe, with which the blood of sacrificed animals was ritually offered in Germanic cult practice, was similarly regarded by the Celts as the all-healing blood-twig. Epilepsy was also treated with mistletoe, since it was believed that this suffering originates in the otherworld.

Since the mistletoe can provide access to the otherworld and to the dead, it is also regarded as a bringer of fertility, because fertility is a gift from the ancestors. For this reason, every thirty years the Celtic Druids performed a ritual cutting of mistletoe on the accession of a newly crowned king to ensure his potency and fruitfulness. The king was considered the husband of the goddess of the land; he was responsible for the fertility of the herds, meadows, and fields. In his *Natural History* (XVI, 95), the Roman civil servant Pliny the Elder (23–79 CE) described the princely ritual whereby "on the sixth day of the moon . . . and after every thirty years of a new generation" the mistletoe, which they call "healing of all things," is cut from a "hard-oak":

> They prepare a ritual sacrifice and banquet beneath [the] tree and
> bring up two white bulls, whose horns are bound for the first time
> on this occasion. A priest arrayed in white vestments climbs the tree

and with a golden sickle cuts down the mistletoe, which is caught in a white cloak. They finally kill the victims, praying to God to render his gift propitious to those upon whom it is bestowed. (Pliny 1945, 551–52)

The slimy mistletoe berries were believed to be semen drops of the heavenly bull, which fertilize the Earth Goddess.

No common peasant or regular herbalist among the Celts would have gone to such efforts to get the mistletoe; the ritual is clearly part of the high culture. This does not mean, however, that the common people did not also apply this cure-all for healing and magic purposes. In European folk medicine, mistletoe is still considered a cure for infertility: a popular traditional cure is to boil three mistletoe twigs in a pint of old white wine with some sugar for three minutes and drink eight days before the onset of the menstrual period; this is claimed to unfailingly cause pregnancy. Maria Treben, who draws on this tradition, states that fresh mistletoe juice can cure a woman's infertility (Treben 2017, 99). Dizziness, epilepsy, tumors, hemorrhages, bloody vomiting, convulsions, menopausal problems, and "bad juices" were also treated with this plant, which the Germans call *Fallkraut* (the fall-herb, traditionally used for falling sickness) and *Heil aller Schäden* (healer of all harms). The sticky, slimy berries were used much less because they are poisonous.

Rudolf Steiner gave the parasitic plant a new therapeutic indication as a cancer remedy. It has become the anticancer drug par excellence in anthroposophic medicine. Experiments confirm that the injected mistletoe extract stimulates the immune system, inhibits growths, and increases killer cells (T-cells) that mature in the thymus. This stimulating effect was probably already recognized by Hippocrates, who allegedly prescribed mistletoe for the treatment of spleen disorders. The spleen, a lymphatic organ, is known to be part of the immune system. "The mistletoe re-adheres the mind, soul, and vitality to the physical body, thus resolving any immunity weakness" (Reinhard 2008, 143).

In Europe, mistletoe still plays a role in folkloric superstitions. Some of the European common names indicate that it is indeed an unusual plant: German *Hexennest* (witch's nest), *Hexenbesen* (witch's broom), *Teufelsast* (devil's branch), *Teufelsbesen* (devil's broom), *Trudennest* (*trud*'s nest; *trud* = "oppressive night spirit"), *Gespensterrute* (ghost rod), *Alpranken* (*Alp*-creeper; *Alp* = "nightmare spirit"), and *Marentake* (nightmare-spirit's twig; Low German *mare*, "nightmare spirit," + *take*, "twig"); and the French *buchon de sorcière* (sorcerer's cork) or *gui des druides* (druids' misteltoe). A mistletoe berry encased in silver and worn as an amulet, or placed in the barn or under the roof, keeps witches and other fiendish astral entities at bay. Cooked in beer, mistletoe is a healing potion for bewitched cattle. If the mistletoe grows on an old hazel tree, it is a sign that one might find buried treasure or even a "hazel worm" beneath it.* Where mistletoe grows, no lightning strikes, and harmful earth rays are mitigated.

Of course, such a magic twig had to be harvested with great care. It was not allowed to be cut off with any ordinary knife; it had to be shot down with an arrow or a stone and caught with the left hand. In any case, it should not touch the earth. The best time to obtain it was under a new moon, when the sun is in Sagittarius, or around St. John's Day, the ancient feast of the sun god (Baldur), who was fatally wounded by a mistletoe arrow.

Like the heart, the mistletoe mediates between the forces of below and above. Dowsers assure me that the mistletoe plant influences the sap of the host trees, making them better able to cope with geomantic or electromagnetic interference fields.

Motherwort
(*Leonurus cardiaca*)

Motherwort, a mint family (Lamiaceae) member, has always been a heart plant—but not in the modern sense. The plant, which in German is called *Herzgespann* (heart-cramps) or *Herzgesperr* (heart-

---

*Folklore has it that whoever finds the "hazel worm"—a white snake with a golden crown—and eats of its flesh will instantly know every healing plant and understand the language of the animals.

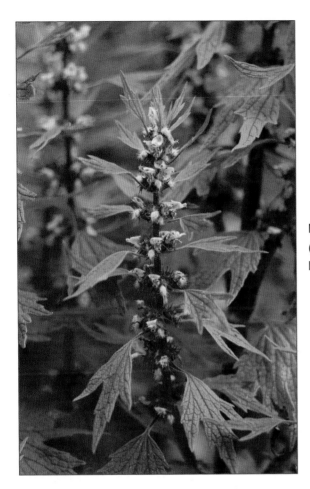

Motherwort
(*Leonurus cardiaca*)
leaves and flowers

lock), terms that describe pressure and anxiety in the chest, is believed to be referring to tension of the "heartbands" (perhaps what we today call the pericardium). In earlier times, tensions in the diaphragm and stomach were also called *Herzgespann* (see "Nervous Heart" on page 15) In the *Gart der Gesundheit* (Garden of Health; Schöffer 1485), a German translation of the Latin natural history encyclopedia *Hortus Sanitatus,* we read:

> This crushed plant and its juice, when used in its purest form, takes away the pain in the heart, and makes the blood well again. This plant is good for an unsteady heart. (Marzell 1943–1979, II:1242)

The root crushed in this manner was placed on the chest. Motherwort is called *Teuichrut* (*Teui*-herb) in Schaffhausen (Switzerland), and it is used when an animal loses its digestive power (*Teui*).

The plant is a native of southeastern Europe and Central Asia but is now found worldwide due to its use as an herbal remedy. Throw-wort, lion's tail, and lion's ear are other names.

Motherwort was used for women's ailments, such as *Mutterweh* (mother's pain—that is, labor pains or uterine problems). For example, we learn from the English herbalist Nicholas Culpeper of the motherwort:

> Venus owns the herb and it is under Leo. There is no better herb to take melancholy vapours from the heart, to strengthen it, and make a merry, cheerful, blithe soul than this herb. It may be kept in a syrup or conserve; therefore the Latins called it Cardiaca. In addition, it makes women joyful mothers of children, and settles their wombs as they should be, therefore we call it Motherwort. It is held to be of much use for the trembling of the heart, and faintings and swoonings; from whence it took the name Cardiaca. The powder thereof, to the quantity of a spoonful, drank in wine, is a wonderful help to women in their sore travail, as also for the suffocating or risings of the mother [uterus], and for these effects, it is likely it took the name of Motherwort with us. It also provokes urine and women's courses, cleanses the chest of cold phlegm, oppressing it, kills worms in the belly. It is of good use to warm and dry up the cold humours, to digest and disperse them that are settled in the veins, joints, and sinews of the body, and to help cramps and convulsions. (Culpeper 1999, 121)

In Saxony, Thuringia, and Lusatia, motherwort was also used against witchcraft.* It was referred to as "enchantment herb" (German *Beschreikraut;* Sorbian *pódrjene zelo*) and placed in the cradle or under

---

*Lusatia (German Lausitz) was a region inhabited by the Sorbs, a West Slavic group.

the pillow of the children if they slept restlessly and were thought to have been bewitched.

Today the medical indications for motherwort are somewhat different. Primarily, it is used in the case of disturbances to the heart's vegetative functions; it has a calming effect on the heart. Second, it is effective—like gypsywort (*Lycopus europaeus*)—in treating an overactive thyroid (hyperthyroidism); and third, it helps treat menopausal symptoms such as hot flashes, anxiety, and nervous restlessness. Motherwort has a contractive effect on the uterus and is antispasmodic; it helps with menstrual disorders (missed or decreasing menstrual periods).

Cardiac glycosides are not present in motherwort, but bitter diterpenes, betaines, flavonoids, caffeic acid derivatives, and triterpenes are. Motherwort is best prepared as a tea and taken over a long period of time (three months is the usual recommendation for a healing tea cure) or taken in the form of a tincture.

Mountain Arnica
(*Arnica montana*)

In the summer, golden-yellow light is reflected in the disc and ray florets of arnica, which grows wild in remote forests and moist meadows throughout Europe. In the United States there are also varities of arnica that can be used in similar ways as European arnica; typically it is *Arnica montana* that is cultivated for medicinal use. Even though it does not avoid moist soil, arnica is completely devoted to the light and the sun. It can be found up to 2,800 meters (9,816 ft.) above sea level. The plant does not like lime soils, and artificial fertilizer makes it disappear.

Arnica is one of the midsummer "flowers of St. John." When the rural women used to gather their plant medicinals in meadows, hedgerows, and forests, arnica flowers were part of the "St. John's bunch" or "solstice bouquet" of herbs collected on the eve of St. John's Day (June 24). These herbs were a way to preserve—usually by drying—part of the light and heat of midsummer to help the people

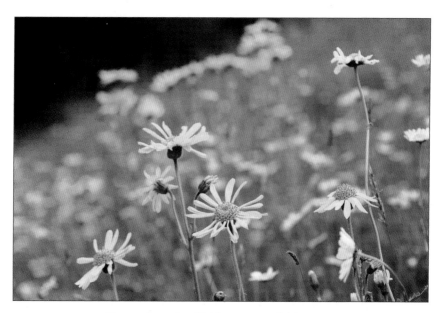

Mountain arnica (*Arnica montana*) blossoms

of northern climates get through the cold wintertime. In addition to *Hypericum perforatum* (St. John's wort), this midsummer bouquet of healing herbs included yarrow, thyme, lady's mantle, and, above all, arnica—also called *Geldblume* (gold flower), *Feuerblume* (fire flower), *Sternenblume* (star flower), *Geel Sankt Johannis Blume* (yellow St. John's flower), and *Sonnwendblüml* (little solstice flower); in Swedish it is called *midsommarblomster* (midsummer flower). As a medicinal plant, in parts of Austria it was called *Kraftwurz* (power wort) or *Kraftrose* (power rose); in Westphalia, *Stoh up un go hen* (Get up and go hence); elsewhere in Germany, *Wundkraut* (wound herb) and *Stichkraut* (stitch herb, which cures stitches in the side).* It is used externally as a tincture for bruises and injuries caused from falling and was therefore also called fall-down herb (*Fallkraut*) in some German dialects. The Christian monks dedicated the plant to St. Lucian of Beauvais. According to legend, this saint, a missionary from Britain who was active in Christianizing the still partly pagan Grisons region

---

*English common names include leopard's bane, wolf's bane, and mountain arnica.

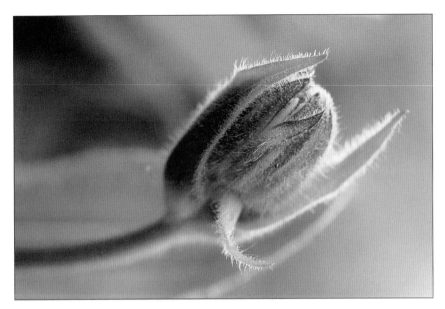

Mountain arnica (*Arnica montana*) bud

(Switzerland) in the fifth and sixth centuries, was thrown into a well and stoned; the severely bruised man was saved by his fellow monks and cured his bruises with arnica. The conclusion is obvious: the consecrated healing plant—St. Lucian's herb (German *Luzianskraut;* French *herbe de Saint-Lucien;* or Dutch *Sint Luciaans wond kruid,* "St. Lucian's wound herb")—relieves bruises, contusions, and the like.

Later, after the Europeans became addicted to tobacco, the powdered leaves of arnica were mixed in with snuff. As a result it became known as a kind of wild tobacco (French *tabac sauvage, tabac Suisse;* Italian *tabacco dei Vosgi*) or snuff (German *Niesblume,* "sneezing flower," because the powder triggers sneezing). This usage is also reflected in several of its English common names: mountain snuff and mountain tobacco.

In Germanic plant classification, it is considered a wolf plant, which is reflected in several of its other common names: *Wolfsgelb* (wolf's yellow), *Wolfsauge* (wolf's eye), and *Wolfsblume* (wolf's flower); an English common name is wolf's bane. Like wolf's milk (euphorbia), monkshood, hemlock, and so on, it is a very poisonous plant—a raging wolf among the herbs. If arnica is ingested, the symptoms include stomach pain, vomiting, an excruciating urge to urinate and defecate (with little voiding), rapid pulse and accelerated breathing, cardiac disorders, severe sweating, dizziness, back and shoulder pain, reduced vision, and irritating sexual agitation. Conrad Gesner, the first botanist to mention arnica (in 1561), tasted two drachmas (1 drachma = 3.75 grams) and wrote the famous last words that the tea had become him very well. An hour later he was dead! The dose had been too high. Externally, the juice can also be highly irritating to the skin and cause hives.

But perhaps the plant's wolf name is not only a reflection of its toxicity. It is quite possible that the name has a connection to ancient pagan midsummer grain and crop rituals. Folklore scholars inform us that, in earlier times, the fertile power of the field was seen as a boisterous grain spirit or vegetation numen.* This was imagined in the form of an old hag (such as the *Kornmuhme* [grain mother] or *Zitzenweib* [teathag], the ancient goddess of growth), a wild sow, a goat (the horned Paleolithic god), or, very frequently, a wolf. Amid the swaying cereal crop in the field, the rye-wolf (*Röggenwolf*) or grain-wolf (*Kornwolf*) was seen roaming furtively through the grain (Bächtold-Stäubli 1987, V:256). If this fertile power, imagined as a wolf, leaves the field, then the grain rots and withers. To keep the grain-wolf in the field, the wolf plant, arnica, which blooms at this time of the year, was planted at the four corners of the field. The grain-wolf was believed to be hiding in the last sheaf of grain, which was cut at the end of the harvest in August. This sheaf was then decorated and solemnly carried to the village. Originally, it was the shamanic priests and priestesses called the *bilwis* who cast their spells to keep the grain-wolf within the fields. They blessed the field and ritually cut a handful of grain—three stalks, respectively—at each corner of the field. After Christianization, these heathen grain priests were transmogrified into destructive sorcerers and witches. In many places the term *Bilwisschnitter* came to be synonymous with wicked grain spirits who ride on a billy goat through the fields or

---

*See footnote on page 145.

cut wild patterns in the grain field with sickles gone amok, make the ears of grain black and sooty (ergot!), and cause other damage.*

Even after these grain shamans had disappeared, arnica continued to play a role in summer solstice customs. For a long time, the agriculturists continued to collect arnica flowers for the St. John's bouquets or put them in the "St. John's bed"—a bed of flowers, originally for the sun god, or Baldur—in which, after Christianization, John the Baptist should rest. In addition, the farmers put bunches of arnica around the edges of the fields on St. John's eve, but now they were to keep away the evil grain spirit (*bilewits*).

Hildegard of Bingen mentioned arnica, which she called *wolfesgelegena* (wolf's lain), not as a medicinal herb but for use in a love spell:

> *Wolfesgelegena* is very hot and has a poisonous heat in it. If a person's skin has been touched with fresh arnica, he or she will burn lustily with love for the person who is afterward touched by the same herb. He or she will be so incensed with love, almost infatuated, and will become a fool. (Hildegard of Bingen 1998, 75)

Hildegard is probably also referring to the ecstatic goings-on at summer solstice, which—as a fertility festival—often took on orgiastic features.

Like other midsummer flowers, such as the elderflower or the linden blossom, which capture the warmth of the sun and, after ingestion, bring heat into the body and cause it to sweat, arnica was also considered a sudorific. For use in this manner, it was boiled in beer. Arnica that was plucked on St. John's eve could be employed as "thunder

---

*The *bilewits* (Germanic *bil*, "miraculous, effective, right, fitting," *wit*, "white" or "knowing"; Dutch *bilwit*; Old English *bilewit*) were white-clad priests with shaggy hair ("Bilwis locks," which today might be called dreadlocks). There seems to be a relationship here to the Celtic Bel and the Germanic Baldur, Phol, or Beldeg (Anglo-Saxon), the sun god in his midsummer guise (Vries 2000, 50; Storl 2000, 28). The Germanic peoples called upon the gods as *bilewit*, the "benevolent ones." After the conversion to Christianity, they transferred the word to Christ as the "spiritual sun," then later to the angels, and finally onto a nature spirit, which was viewed more and more negatively as time went on.

flower" (*Donnerblume*)—a protection against stormy midsummer weather, lightning, heavy thunderstorms, and hail, which threatened the ripening grain. To this end the arnica bunch was hung in the Herrgottswinkel of the house or under the roof, or burned as incense along with the saying:

> *Steck Arnica an, steck Arnica an,*
> *dass sich das Wetter scheiden kann.*

> Burn, arnica, burn,
> So bad weather won't return.

From the brief sketch I have presented here, it is clear arnica, with its light-nature, has a relation to the life-sustaining grain and the sun, the heart of the macrocosm. Like the sun, which keeps the cycle of the year and the natural water cycle (evaporation, cloud formation, rain) in motion, this small flower of the sun helps the human heart and the circulatory system—for example, with poor blood circulation of the fine vessels or with aging heart and coronary disease (with or without angina pectoris). A tea made from the flowers of arnica, drunk slowly and swallowed, or five to ten drops of arnica tincture, has a stimulating effect on the tired heart (of course, this poisonous plant should only be administered internally by a medical professional). Arnica acts fast—faster than hawthorn, for example—and is intended for short-term application. In contrast to hawthorn, high doses of arnica are dangerous, leading to dizziness, tachycardia, arrhythmia, and eventual collapse, or even death. For a long-lasting, curative treatment, one should instead use hawthorn tea (Weiss 2001, 228). Incidentally, arnica contains neither alkaloids nor glycosides but instead essential oils, carotenoids, and flavonoids.

In his latter years, the German poet Goethe repeatedly resorted to the plant. In February to March of 1823, the seventy-four-year-old writer had to spend nine days and nights sitting in his armchair due to severe shortness of breath and heart pains, enduring the "dreadful miasmas" that had burdened him "for three thousand years."

He literally had a "broken heart," after young Ulrike von Levetzow had renounced his love. He viewed the doctors and their arts, as always, with skepticism. It was the old practice of leeching and, above all, arnica, which helped him out of the crisis (Nager 1992, 35). Enthusiastically, he then paid homage to "this splendid plant that belongs to the lofty heights of primordial rock, that grows at the steps of the gods' thrones!" In flowery language he described its growth and opening of the blossom:

> It bursts its tight confinement, yellow-red whirls of fire stand into the light of the St. John's sun. What piquancy, what fragrance! . . . What it smells like, how can I express it? I would like to call it "healing force." . . . In every way, energy is piled into the arnica plant. Just the memory of it pours fire-streams around my heart. But force is paired here with a delicate form. Nothing brittle, nothing hard opposes the creative power of the sky; young and fresh with vitality, the sun-god chose this flower. Gaze upon the blossom—how it opens, how it dissolves in light, in the glow of the sun. . . . Here is the plant of rapid healing, of powerful decision. If harms have been forcibly done to you from the outside—bumps, blows, cutting wounds—in this plant wondrous help for you is at hand. The vital forces stream, the pulse strengthens, the heart becomes emboldened; what lost its way as a bloody rupture, as vascular tumor, remembers the right path. Muscles and tendons become taut; the body, injured and damaged, rights itself—but the nervous system, which is difficult to heal, does so thoroughly as well. The organic indignation at the damage we have suffered, which we call pain, eases and ebbs away. . . . I felt when life and death began to war within me, that the troops of life, with this flower on their banner, forced a breakthrough: for the hostile, stagnant, and deadly depressing enemy, they prepared its Austerlitz.*
> Rejuvenated in my recovery, I praise arnica most—and it is, indeed,

---

*The phrase "prepared its Austerlitz" is an idiom that refers to a decisive 1805 battle in Austerlitz in Moravia, where Napoleon inflicted a defeat on the Austrian and Russian armies.

only nature praising itself, truly inexhaustible nature that produces such a flower. (Goethe 1948, 249–50)

Periwinkle
(*Vinca minor*)

Periwinkle, a blue-flowering dogbane (Apocynaceae family) plant that likes to grow in shady, enchanted places, in cemeteries or old castle ruins, was always considered a magical herb. It is native to central and southern Europe, as well as the Caucasus and southwestern Turkey. In the United States, it is considered an invasive plant, though it is also cherished by some as a lovely ground cover. Vinca, the Latin name, comes from *vincire*, "bind, enwrap, tie, shackle" and "transmit, obligate, ban, enchant." In the *Gart der Gesundheit* (Garden of Health) one reads:

> *Syngrün, Berwinica:**. . . The devil has no power over anyone who has this plant on their person. No witchcraft can come into the house where this herb is hung over the front door. With the help of the herb, one can determine in whom an evil spirit dwells. It works best when it is consecrated with other herbs on the Day of Our Lady.[†] (Schöffer 1485)

Nicholas Culpeper, who put the periwinkle under Venus's rule, wrote: "Venus owns this herb, and saith, That the leaves eaten by man and wife together, cause love between them" (Culpeper 1999, 139). For

---

*Pliny called the plant *vinca pervinca,* and from the latter word derive the old German names such as *Berwunca* and *Berwinkel* and the English name periwinkle. The old German name *Singrun* (*Syngrün*) is composed of *sin-,* "everlasting" + *grün,* "green," meaning that the leaves never wilt; the modern German name for the plant, *Immergrün,* has the same sense: "ever-green."
[†]The Feast of the Assumption of Mary, August 15, is also the day of the Mary's herb consecration (*Mariawürzweih*), meant for all healing herbs. This custom of blessing wild herbs and flowers was instituted by the church as far back as the tenth century.

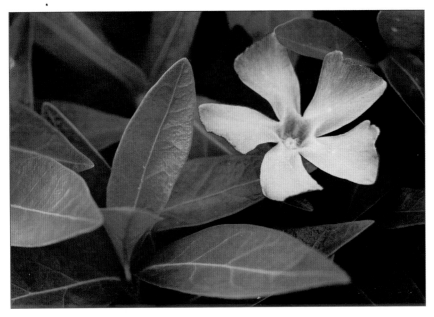

Periwinkle (*Vinca minor*) blossom

Christians, periwinkle was a symbol of eternal fidelity, and its sky-blue flowers were considered a sign of the Virgin Mary.

In the old herbals it is used to treat nosebleeds, diarrhea, toothache, poisonous animal bites, headaches (a "devil" in the head), memory problems, and dizziness. Back in the nineteenth century, country folk hung a small bag of periwinkle roots around the necks of their children so that they would be always attentive and clever at school (Zerling 2007, 124).

Today, despite the negative monograph of the Commission E,* periwinkle is used in Germany to increase blood flow to the heart and brain. The indole alkaloid vincamine reduces blood pressure, relaxes the autonomic nervous system, and increases the oxygen uptake of the brain. Periwinkle is appropriate after strokes and minor brain injuries, as well as for dizziness, presbycusis, and tinnitus. In this sense, it has a similar effect to ginkgo.

---

*See footnote on page 169.

Scotch Broom
(*Cytisus scoparius,* formerly *Sarothamnus scoparius*)

Scotch broom, also called common broom, is a pale-yellow flowering member of the legume family (Fabaceae), which likes to grow on sandy heaths or at the edges of oak forests. It is native to central and western Europe and is considered an invasive species in the United States, Australia, New Zealand, Canada, and India.

For the Celts, this plant that blooms lavishly in May was a symbol of the victorious young sun god Belenos who weds the goddess at the May full moon. In the medieval flower language, Scotch broom represented humility and humiliation. In the twelfth century, when Geoffrey V, Count of Anjou, took his crusade vow, as a sign of his humble submission to the power of the church he removed the proud plume from his

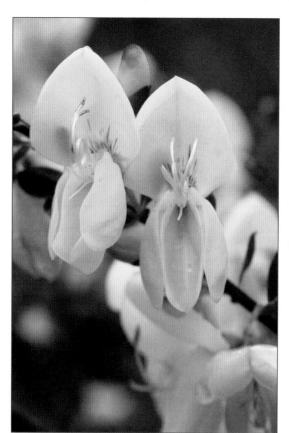

Scotch broom
(*Cytisus scoparius*)
blossoms

helmet and replaced it with a sprig of the common broom. His family epithet, Plantagenet, derives from this (Old French *plante genest,* "broom plant"). The related gorse (*Ulex europaeus*), with its nasty thorns, was, by contrast, regarded in the Middle Ages as a symbol of sin and hellfire.

In folklore of the British Isles, broom is considered one of the nine plants that are especially dear to the elves. Anglo-Saxon healers and the Welsh Myddfai physicians used this diuretic plant mainly for dropsy and to "open" the spleen, liver, or kidneys. In the Middle Ages, a brew of the boiled sprig tips was used as a blood purifier for help with rheumatism, gout, and jaundice.

Only in the modern times did broom come into use as a medicinal plant for heart problems. Broom contains no glycosides but does contain flavonoids and, above all, quinolizidine alkaloids, which, similarly to nicotine, act as a ganglion blocker, hindering and reducing heart conduction. It is appropriate for tachycardia arrhythmia, when the heart beats unevenly, skips, or makes extra beats, as well as in atrial fibrillation. Broom is not only supportive against disorders in the regulation of the circulatory system, but it also helps with low blood pressure and improves the venous return of the blood.

UNIVERSAL CARDIAC PHYTOTHERAPEUTICS

Arjun Tree
(*Terminalia arjuna*)

The arjun or myrobalene tree belongs to the white mangrove family (Combretaceae). The mighty tree is at home in the monsoon forests of South Asia. In Indian culture it bears the name of the hero of the *Mahabharata* epic, Arjuna. This epic tells the story of a bloody struggle between two related royal clans. The noble warrior Arjuna and his brothers were faced with the choice of having the power and glory of the world placed at their feet or contentment with god's (Vishnu's) presence; similar to the Christian dilemma of having the power of the

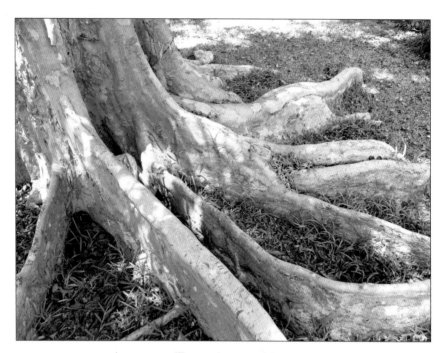

Arjun tree (*Terminalia arjuna*) lower trunk

world at your disposal or serving Christ. This is a choice every human soul must make in life—the choice between the path of worldly glory and that of the heart. Arjuna chose the path of the heart, while his hostile, power-hungry relatives chose the path of the world. After his decision, his own divine Self approached him. But Arjuna did not recognize it, for it had assumed the form of his servant Krishna, the driver of his chariot, just before the great battle that was to be waged between the hosts of the warring clans. Arjuna was depressed, tormented by his conscience—he was unwilling to fight, as he did not want to kill and incur guilt. Then his young charioteer turned to him and made him see his true unfathomable divine nature. He calmed the reluctant warrior, reminded him of the immortality of the soul, and exhorted him to do his karmic duty. After that, Krishna (representing the divine Self) steered the horses (representing the senses) safely through the fray (representing daily life) and led Arjuna to victory.

In relation to our subject, one could interpret this story from the *Bhagavad Gita*—the most well-known part of the *Mahabharata*—in

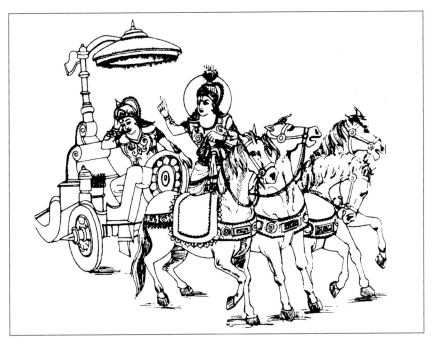

Krishna and Arjuna

the following way. Whoever allows the divine to enter his soul will also have a healthy heart; he who pursues the false luster of the world and is driven by the lust for power and wealth, or by sexual lust, will find his heart in danger; it will lose its rhythm and break down. If that is the case, then the arjun tree can help. Arjun is a cardiotonic that has been documented to have been mentioned in early Sanskrit texts (2700 BCE) (Bakhru 1993, 25).

Arjun tree bark is indicated for coronary heart disease (Sanskrit *hridroga*), tachycardia, angina, heart failure, myocardial infarction, and high blood pressure (Zoller and Nordwig 1997, 501). Its effect is cardiotonic and antihypertensive: the heart muscle is better nourished; the contraction increases and at the same time the frequency decreases. The powder or decoction of the calcium-rich, silver-white bark of the tree is used as a heart drug. Arjun powder can be taken to strengthen the heart muscles after a heart attack or as a preventive measure. In Ayurvedic medicine, the three fundamental principles (*tridoshas*)—*vata*, "wind"; *kapha*, "phlegm"; and *pitta*, "fire"—which have a formative effect in the human microcosm as well as in nature, are considered in relation to health issues. With each person, depending on his or her nature, one of the *doshas* is in the foreground. Diseases also manifest in these three forms. If the heart disease is of a *vata* nature, then the powder should be mixed with clarified butter (ghee); if it has a fiery *pitta* nature, then it is taken with milk; if it is *kapha* in nature, then the bark powder should be mixed with honey or pepper (Dash 1995, 71).

New clinical research has revealed that the medicament in arjun is an antioxidant; it improves the endothelial tissue (inner lining of the blood vessels), even in smokers; it makes the blood more fluent and helps to regulate blood pressure; and it causes LDL cholesterol to be metabolized more quickly by the liver. Triterpene glycosides are responsible for the effect; coenzyme Q-10 protects against heart attack and lowers blood pressure; and flavonoids act as antioxidants.

The giant arjun tree is, of course, also a sacred tree. One of the last twenty-four Buddhas in Sri Lanka is said to have found enlightenment under an arjun. The following legend is told on the subcontinent about the origin of the tree:

The king of the forest tree spirits had two sons. One day, when they had drunk too much intoxicating wine, they stripped off their clothes and chased after heavenly maidens. Laughing and howling, they ran past an old sage without greeting him properly. Then the yogi cursed the naked youths and turned them into arjun trees. As punishment, boats and tools are now made from their wooden bodies, and leather is tanned with their skins (bark). However, the people who fell these trees are charitable. The night before cutting down the trees, they say prayers and offer them flowers and incense. They sprinkle holy water on the logs and rub the ax blades with butter and honey; and before carving ordinary things out of their wood, they first carve small statues of the gods. (Patnaik 1993, 79)

Coffee
(*Coffea arabica*)

A good coffee must be as hot as the kisses of a girl on the first day, as sweet as her love on the third day, and as black as her mother's curses when she finds out about it.

OLD ASIAN COFFEEHOUSE PROVERB

Everyone is familiar with coffee, or at least with the roasted coffee bean. Brewed from the seeds of this member of the madder family (Rubiaceae), originally from the Ethiopian highlands, coffee lifts the mood and makes the drinker slightly euphoric—a trait already appreciated by the Muslim Sufi dervishes. In the middle of the seventeenth century, the first coffeehouses opened in Italy. The beverage came to central Europe after the Ottoman Turks, who had besieged Vienna for several months, were routed by the forces of the Holy Roman Empire

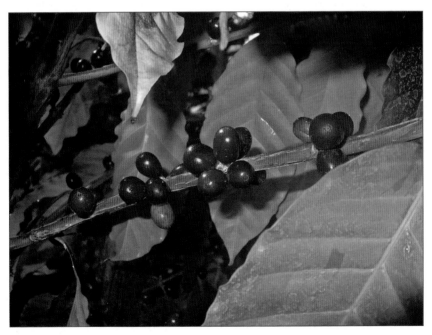

Coffee (*Coffea arabica*) leaves and fruit

at the Battle of Vienna in 1683. Among the many supplies they left behind were bags of coffee beans. Most people assumed it was camel fodder. One clever entrepreneur, however, knew what he was dealing with and soon started up the first Viennese coffeehouse. The bitter black brew became the fuel for the intellectuals of the Enlightenment. Newspapers and encyclopedias were written under its influence. The coffeehouses were home to heated conversations, which gave rise to the revolutionary ideas that called the old feudal system into question. There were even doctors who proclaimed coffee to be a quasi-panacea and sent their patients to a café rather than the pharmacy (Müller 1982, 680).

From the start, voices of warning could also be heard. The diuretic drink was said to dry out the kidneys, nerves, and brain. The great doctor Albrecht von Haller (1708–1777) said that coffee causes "the blood to heat up." It disrupts the nerves, and ultimately leads to general drowsiness and impotence. A children's song of the times warns:

> *C-A-F-F-E-E,*
> *trink nicht zu viel Kaffee,*
> *nicht für Kinder ist der Türkentrank, schwächt die*
> *Nerven,*
> *macht dich blass und krank.*
> *Sei doch kein Muselmann,*
> *der das nicht lassen kann.*

> C-o-f-f-e-e,
> do not drink too much coffee,
> the Turkish drink is not for kids,
> it weakens the nerves,
> makes you pale and wan.
> So don't be like a Mussulman,
> who cannot give it up.

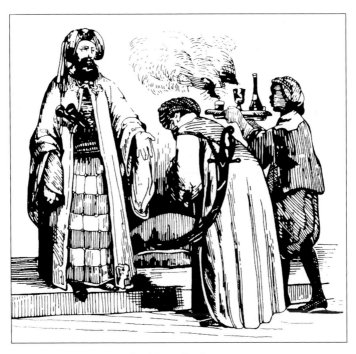

Arabic coffeehouse

Even today, the jury is still out regarding the effects of coffee. The purine alkaloid caffeine accelerates the pulse and can affect cardiac output by reducing diastolic relaxation. Overdoses irritate the gastric mucosa and cause heart palpitations, hemorrhoids, agitation, and insomnia. Time and again, it has been alleged that coffee heightens the risk of a heart attack.

In the meantime, however, numerous studies show that coffee does not cause heart attacks or strokes (Pollmer and Warmuth 2003, 174). On the contrary, caffeine has a stimulating effect on the cerebral cortex and directly on the heart muscle, whose tonus it increases. Therefore, coffee is prescribed for shock, circulatory disorders, and circulatory insufficiency. It also improves kidney circulation and, as a result, urination. Only patients with myocardial infarction, high blood pressure, and thyroid hyperfunction should avoid the drink.

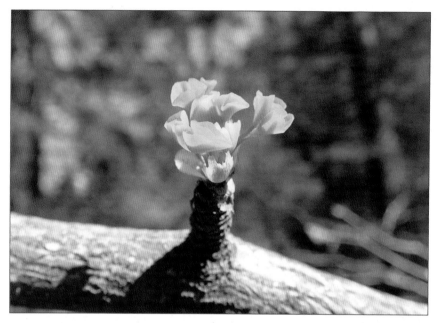

Ginkgo (*Ginkgo biloba*) shoot

Ginkgo
(*Ginkgo biloba*)

The ginkgo tree, also called the maidenhair tree, is ancient. It is a living fossil. It was already growing here on earth in the Mesozoic era, 300 million years ago, and was—like other gymnosperms—a part of the dinosaurs' diet. Because the fan-like leaves were known only from imprints in anthracite, it was believed that the plant, like the giant reptiles, had long since died out. But then a German doctor, Engelbert Kämpfer, who was accompanying a Dutch legation, discovered the tree in a Buddhist monastery in Japan in 1691. In 1712, he published the first scientific treatise on the tree, and in 1737 he planted the first ginkgo in the Dutch city of Utrecht. Since the eighteenth century ginkgos have been keenly planted as park trees in Europe. Goethe was enthusiastic about the tree and dedicated a poem to it that begins with the following lines:

Dieses Baumes Blatt, der vom Osten
Meinem Garten anvertraut,

Giebt geheimen Sinn zu kosten,
Wie's den Wissenden erbaut.

In my garden's care and favour
From the East this tree's leaf shows
Secret sense for us to savour
And uplifts the one who knows.

(GOETHE 1998, 120)

Today, ginkgo is planted mainly in cities because it is particularly resistant to air pollution, car exhaust, cell-phone radiation, mildew, viruses, and parasites. Its resilience was demonstrated in Hiroshima when the atomic bomb was dropped in 1945, pulverizing the city center and wiping out all life in the vicinity. The following spring, not far from ground zero, one saw a miracle: out of the blackened stump of a ginkgo tree, there grew a tender young shoot. This shoot, which has since become a tall tree, became a symbol of hope for all of humanity.

The wild ginkgo has practically disappeared. Buddhist and Taoist monks in East Asia, however, guarded the living fossil in their temple forests. With incense sticks and rituals, they worshipped the tree—which can grow more than one hundred feet high and achieve an age of 2,000 years—as a symbol of long life and wisdom. Chinese monks chewed the leaves to keep their spirits lively and reach old age. These monks probably saved the tree from extinction.

The ginkgo, whose historical development can be situated between tree ferns and conifers, is dioecious—in other words, there are male and female trees. The female fruit is the color and size of a small plum. These "eggs" are fertilized not only by airborne pollen (spermatozoa) while hanging on the branches—if the fruit have fallen from the tree to the ground, they can still be fertilized by male spermatozoa, which "swim" on the moist soil surface toward the eggs, unite with them, and a new ginkgo embryo begins to grow.

In East Asia, the fruits—the Chinese call them *yin xing,* "silver

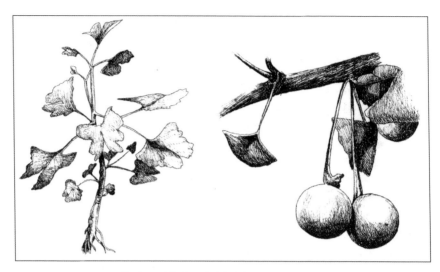

Ginkgo (*Ginkgo biloba*) leaves and fruits

apricots"—are collected diligently because the kernels are cherished as a delicacy, roasted or boiled. However, they are toxic if eaten raw. The fleshy outer layer must be removed to get to the core, which exudes an unpleasant odor after maturity. The scent has been variously described as reminiscent of rancid butter, dog poop, a billy goat, or vomit. For this reason, in the West one rarely encounters female specimens of the ginkgo. One of the tree's many Chinese names is *kung sun shu,* "Grandfather-Grandchild Tree." It takes thirty to forty years to become sexually mature, which means that a benevolent grandfather must plant the tree for his grandchildren so that they can enjoy the delicacy.

The ginkgo seeds are classified as officinal in traditional Chinese medicine (TCM). They support the lungs and help with a chronic cough, asthma, and lung mucus. Meanwhile, it has been discovered that the ginkgolic acid it contains can inhibit the growth of tuberculosis bacteria. The seeds are also used to treat vaginal discharge, cloudy urine, spermatorrhoea, and incontinence (Hempen and Fischer 2007, 840). In contrast to Western phytotherapy, the leaves are rarely used in China.

In Europe, the tea or tincture of ginkgo leaves has become one of the most widely used plant medicines. The areas of indication are peripheral arterial occlusive disease (circulatory disorders of the external tissues), brain ischemia (lack of blood supply to the brain), heart failure due to old age, dizziness, and tinnitus. The active substances are flavonol glycosides and terpenes (ginkgolides), which help the blood remain fluent, reducing the risk of thrombosis and strokes. They are anti-inflammatory and antioxidant (as radical scavengers). Ginkgo preparations should not be taken with other blood thinners or with MAO inhibitors.

Indian Snakeroot
(*Rauvolfia serpentina*)

Also called devil pepper or serpentine wood, the snakeroot bush is a plant in the dogbane family (Apocynaceae), which thrives in the foothills of the Himalayas as well as throughout India and East Asia. The bitter-tasting root of the plant, known in Hindi as *chota chand* (little moon) and in Sanskrit as *sarpagandha* (fragrance of the serpent), has been used in ayurveda and Indian folk medicine for at least four thousand years to treat hives, high fever, constipation, epilepsy, insanity, insomnia, intestinal parasites, high blood pressure, and sexual

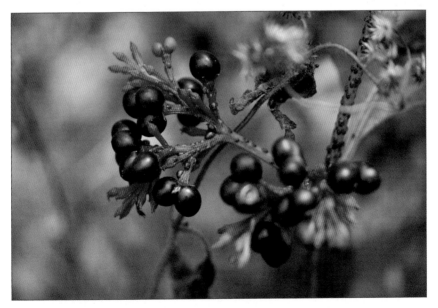

Indian snakeroot (*Rauvolfia serpentina*), also known as devil pepper

overexcitement. Women used it as a labor medicine to accelerate child-birth. Bites from snakes, scorpions, centipedes, and insects are treated with snakeroot. Snakeroot is an effective remedy for mental illnesses that manifest themselves in anxiety and aggression. It calms the mind and improves the *ojas* (life energy). Rauvolfia was Mahatma Ghandi's drug. The Indian freedom fighter drank his cup of rauvolfia tea every night to get some rest. His mass movement of passive, nonviolent resistance to the British colonial authorities would have been inconceivable without the help of the snakeroot plant.

In the West, the molecular components were identified and analyzed in the laboratory. In 1952, the chemist Emil Schletter isolated the main active ingredient, the alkaloid reserpine. It was put on the market as a new miracle drug for lowering blood pressure. But it was not long before alarming reports began to accumulate. The treatment with the pure alkaloid brought many patients into manic-depressive states, which occasionally led to suicide. Prolonged use also seemed to lead to Parkinson's disease. With usage of the whole plant, in which not only reserpine but another 160 different alkaloids are present, such side effects are unknown. Indian mothers even give toddlers soothing *chota chand* tea to drink without any problems.

In the 1970s, however, it was not only the pure alkaloid reserpine that was made available only by prescription but the herbal tea as well. Today, the precious medicinal plant—whose export once provided income to many poor Indian farmers—is no longer available and has been replaced by various dubious synthetic drugs from the pharmaceutical laboratory.

It is simplistic, reductionistic thinking that seeks to reduce the efficacy of a medicinal plant to an essential, isolated agent. These active substances—which are usually alkaloids—can be described as almost moribund molecular complexes that have "fallen out of the life-stream" and been deposited in special cells, with the result having rather toxic effects. Such substances are relatively easy to extract and refine; they can be stored for long periods and synthetically replicated. The pure substances are simple to administer—orally or hypodermically—and are therefore more marketable (and more profitable) than the actual herbs (Storl 2006b, 18). According to Rudolf Fritz Weiss, it is not a single substance but the interaction of the many alkaloids in *Rauvolfia serpentina* that is important. Using the overall complex—in other words, the whole plant—improves physical tolerance and mitigates the risk of hypersensitivity (Weiss 2001, 210). Reserpine is to rauvolfia as caffeine is to coffee, or cocaine to the coca leaf (Weil 2000, 124).

Indian snakeroot lowers high blood pressure by expanding the peripheral vessels and slowing the heart rate. It affects the control center in the diencephalon, which regulates blood pressure. The medicinal plant can also be used to treat psychosomatic heart disease and the associated dizziness and feeling of tightness in the chest. According to Rudolf Fritz Weiss, Indian snakeroot is the most effective among the herbal remedies for the treatment of hypertension. He suggests a curative use of the whole plant in small and medium doses. If coronary damage is present at the same time, the drug can also be combined with hawthorn preparations. Weiss concluded that *Rauvolfia serpentina* is the mildest of the hypotensive agents and one of the most valuable (Weiss 2001, 213).

Jiaogulan
(*Gynostemma pentaphyllum*)

Jiaogulan, also known as five-leaf ginseng, poor man's ginseng, miracle grass, fairy herb, sweet tea vine, gospel herb, and southern ginseng, is native to the mountainous region of south-central China (Guangxi and Sichuan regions). There it is much used by the poor rural population. The Chinese government census in the 1970s showed that life expectancy in these areas is particularly high with a disproportionately high number of centenarians. The statistical longevity of the people in the region aroused the interest of the Chinese Academy of Scientific Medicine. The influence of hereditary factors, climate, nutrition, and other factors was investigated. The inhabitants themselves explained their good health was due to drinking the wild-growing *xiancao* ("herb of immortality" or "twisting blue plant"). The natives claimed that

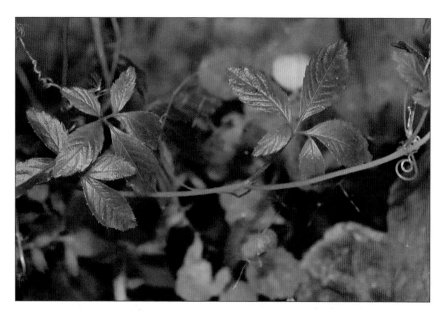

Jiaogulan (*Gynostemma pentaphyllum*) leaves

the tea, which otherwise plays hardly any role at all in official TCM, increased their vitality. In 1978, a group of sixteen scientists headed by Prof. Jialiu Liu researched the plant and documented its effects in about three hundred studies.

In Japan, the plant's name is *amachazuru* (*ama*, "sweet" + *cha*, "tea" + *zuru*, "vine"). Japanese researchers came across this member of the Cucurbitaceae family in their search for alternatives to problematic artificial (low-calorie) sweeteners. The plant has a natural sweetness but is far from being suitable as a sugar substitute. In the 1980s the Japanese undertook intensive chemical composition analyses. They documented eighty-two saponins (gypenosides), which are like the panaxosides (ginsenosides) of ginseng (*Panax ginseng*), as well as trace elements, amino acids, polysaccharides, and vitamins.

In the United States, the newly discovered herb became fashionable as an antiaging plant in the wellness and alternative medicine movement. The book *Jiaogulan: China's "Immortality" Herb* by Michael Blumert and Prof. Jialiu Lui (2012) contributed to this success.

In the book, the following properties are attributed to the plant:

- It keeps the blood pressure within a normal range; the plant acts, like ginseng, as an adaptogen, which means that high blood pressure is lowered and low blood pressure is raised.
- Jiaogulan has an antioxidant effect by stimulating the body's own enzyme superoxide dismutase (SOD).
- As a cardiac tonic it improves the pumping performance of the heart and the general circulation.
- It lowers blood lipid levels, especially LDL levels and triglycerides.
- By counteracting platelet clumping, it prevents thrombosis, stroke, and heart attack.
- It increases the activity of white blood cells and thereby strengthens the immune system (important after radiological or chemotherapeutic treatments).
- It contains the tumor-inhibiting glycoside ginsenoside Rh2.
- The adaptogenic action of the gypenosides improves stress tolerance. It calms the nerves.
- It improves capillary and myocardial blood flow.
- Side effects are not known.

Poison Rope
(*Strophanthus* spp.)

More than forty species of the genus *Strophanthus* are native to the tropical forests of Africa and South Asia. *Strophantus* means "twisted flower" (from Greek *stropha,* "twisted" + *ánthos,* "flower"). The Boers of South Africa call this dogbane plant *gifttou* ("poison dew" or "poison rope"). The names are fitting because the latex that all the shrubs of this genus have is extremely poisonous. The African forest dwellers produce arrow poisons (*kombe, waabaayo, kuna,* etc.) from the seeds, which can bring even the most powerful animals—elephants, buffaloes, and hippos—down in a very short time. The life of many a Portuguese mercenary, slaver, or missionary ended in a hail of just such poison darts. The poison, the alkaloid strophanthin, is stronger

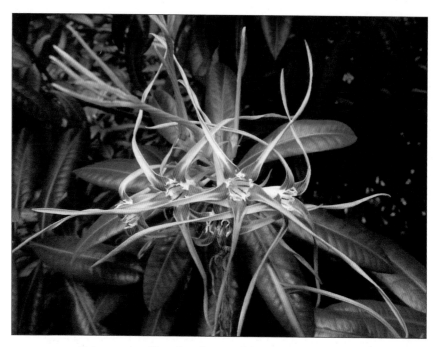

Poison rope (*Strophanthus* spp.) leaves and blossoms

than any snake venom. There are no known antidotes, according to
the research. (African medicine men say they know antidotes, but
they keep them secret).

For the Africans, this dogbane plant, with which they procure
meat and keep their enemies at bay, is a sacred plant. They say a
deity—or the spirit of a leopard or lion—revealed it to them. The
Wilé from Burkina Faso say that it was the little people, the dwarves,
who instructed them in its application. Long ago, a hunter got lost
in pursuit of a porcupine deep in the jungle. For three days and
three nights he wandered around before he collapsed in exhaustion.
Suddenly he heard screaming and the noise of war drums. Frightened,
he saw dangerous-looking, long-haired dwarves coming out of a cave,
followed by a herd of porcupines. The spirits, which were armed with
clubs and knives, surrounded him and threatened him with death—
for the humans had always mistreated and displaced the little people,
and now they wanted to exact revenge on him. But he took courage, told of his mishap, and pled for mercy. Then the spirits of the

mountain consulted with each other and finally said: "We will give you protection, and if you are good and sincere, we will teach you much of our knowledge about curing diseases, snakebites, and poisoning, and which healing herbs to gather to counter poisons, and other antidotes." The hunter followed the pygmies into the cave of the mountain and learned many things, including the production of poisoned arrows from *yabé* (strophantus). Over time, however, he became increasingly sad, as he was homesick. After seven years, seven months, and seven nights and days, the dwarves sent him back to his village. There he became known for his knowledge of the art of healing and poison preparation, but he was also feared. He taught his sons, and the magic knowledge lives on to this day (Neuwinger 1998, 149).

The plant and its seeds are treated with great care. Whoever wants to plant the poisonous shrub must first sacrifice a black chicken to the forest spirits. The clan or village elder then provides the necessary seeds. Early in the morning at the first cock's crow, this person goes into the forest and digs holes; three seeds are placed in each of them. When putting in the seeds, he must turn his back to the east—the east is the direction of life, but this concerns a deadly plant—and close his eyes. If he keeps his eyes open, he will go blind when the seeds germinate, or at the latest, when the twisting plant bears the first fruits.

Many rules and taboos surround the preparation of the poison. For example, the practitioner must not touch a woman of childbearing age, have sexual intercourse, or speak to an unclean person while working with the plant. He must invoke the ancestors, banish evil sorcerers from the circle, and sacrifice a chicken. The way the staggering and dying bird finally falls serves as an oracle. The bubbling brew from the poison seeds is potentized with other ingredients, such as heads of venomous snakes, decayed flesh, scorpions, and so on (Neuwinger 1998, 150).

Dr. John Kirk discovered the cardiac efficacy of the seed by accident in 1859. He was a member of the jungle expedition (1858–1864) with David Livingstone. During the arduous journey, he fell ill with a tropical infection, which caused disturbing, stabbing pains in the heart area. One day, while brushing his teeth, he noticed to his surprise that the pain was suddenly gone. His pulse and racing heart had calmed down. Inspecting his toothbrush closely, he saw that one of the strophanthus seeds, which he had thoughtlessly stored in his toiletries, had stuck between the bristles of his toothbrush. He was startled because he knew it was a notorious dart poison. Would his heart come to a standstill, like a poisoned elephant? However, his heart remained calm, beating evenly.

Upon his return to England, Dr. Kirk related his strange experience while brushing his teeth. The Scottish physician and pharmacologist Thomas Frazer then (1872) set out to isolate an amorphous, water-soluble glycoside from strophanthus seeds. Other chemists after that looked at the substance and recognized its digitalis-like effect: the pulsation frequency is reduced; diastole—the rhythmic expansion of the heart right before a new contraction—becomes larger and longer, and systole becomes stronger; the blood vessels of the viscera contract, while at the same time the brain and kidney vessels expand. Small amounts of strophanthus stimulate the smooth muscle tissue and the heart. After 1904, the substance was available as a pure substance for oral administration.

The German country doctor Albert Fraenkel first seriously treated heart patients with it about this time. He was very successful and came to believe that strophanthin is best administered intravenously. He also recognized that strophanthin helps where digitalis fails. Foxglove intolerance can occur in patients who take it over a long period because the active ingredients accumulate until symptoms of poisoning arise. Strophanthus glycoside (strophanthin), however, has a lower adhesiveness and is eliminated from the heart muscle after six hours. The risk of a cumulative effect is therefore much lower. But perhaps it is not just the accumulation that becomes a problem with digitalis; it is also likely that the foxglove derivatives themselves cause pathological changes in the heart muscle tissue. Such damage does not occur with strophanthin (Schmidsberger 1990, 53). The two cardiac glycosides are similar only in terms of their effectiveness on the pumping deficiency of the heart. Strophanthin is particularly suited for paresthesia that results from an oxygen deficiency in the heart cells. In acute cases strophanthin is mainly administered intravenously. Meanwhile, more and more doctors prescribe oral preparations to prevent the development of cardiac muscle damage due to the cells' oxygen deficiency (Schmidsberger 1990, 167).

In short, strophanthin can substantially prevent angina pectoris attacks by improving the circulation in the heart muscle and brain. Strophanthin increases oxygen energy conversion, improves the flow of red blood cells through the capillaries, accelerates the oxidation of acids, and raises the pH in the heart muscle within a short time. Strophanthin has a relaxing effect on the autonomic nervous system and reduces the stress hormones in the blood and heart muscle. It lowers blood pressure, improves heart performance, and prevents heart hypertrophy. Strophantus thus exhibits the qualities of a whole host of the now common individual drugs, which it could possibly even replace—such as, for example, calcium antagonists, blood-circulation promoters, beta-blockers, antihypertensives, aspirin, anti-inflammatory drugs, and nitro preparations (Petry and Schaefer 2007, 47). Rolf-Jürgen Petry and Hans Schaefer, the authors of the excellently researched book *Die Lösung des Herzinfarkt-Problems durch Strophanthin* (The Solution of the Heart-Attack Problem with Strophanthin), from where this information has been taken, are convinced that academic medicine clearly misjudges strophanthin. They find fault with the supposed low and uncertain absorption of strophanthin. In cardiac medicine today, digitalis (digoxin) advocates and strophantus enthusiasts are in opposing camps. For the latter, there is no doubt that with the help of this African plant, a world without heart attacks could become a reality.

Yellow Oleander
(*Thevetia peruviana*)

The yellow oleander is a plant from the dogbane family (Apocynaceae), which is native to tropical Mexico and Central America and whose leaves resemble the related rose laurel (oleander). In German, it is also

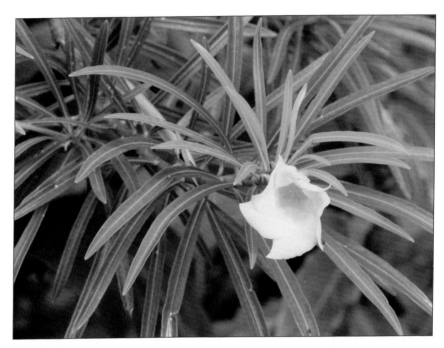

Yellow oleander (*Thevetia peruviana*) leaves and blossom

called *Schellenbaum* (clapper tree) because the indigenous peoples used the hard-shelled seedpod rattles in their dances. The seeds are highly toxic and eight to ten are fatal to humans. In many places, the powder is used in pest control. Indigenous peoples in the Caribbean used the latex of the plant to produce arrow poisons or for poison fishing. In India, where the shrub is planted for ornamentation, Hindus and Buddhists like to use the yellow flower as a flower offering in their rituals of worship (*puja*).

The plant contains heart-effective cardenolide glycosides, which are applicable for cardiac insufficiency and aging heart. They act quickly after ingestion and do not accumulate in the tissue—that is, they have a low cumulative effect (Schönfelder and Schönfelder 2004, 444).

Afterword

The Chinese political reformer and Confucian scholar Zhang Zhidong (1837–1909) made the following remark in his study guide, *Quanxuepian* (Exhortation to Learning, 1898):

> Chinese science is the science of the internal; European science is the science of the external. The aim of Chinese science is to regulate the human heart, while European science is only attuned to the needs of outer life.

A small dose of such Chinese philosophy would certainly be good for us in the West!

REFERENCES

Ammon, Hermann P. T., ed. 2004. *Hunnius Pharmazeutisches Wörterbuch.* Berlin: De Gruyter.

Bächtold-Stäubli, Hanns, ed. 1987. *Handwörterbuch des deutschen Aberglaubens.* 10 vols. Berlin: De Gruyter.

Bakhru, H. K. 1993. *Herbs that Heal.* New Delhi and Bombay: Orient.

Baldwin, William J. 2003. *Healing Lost Souls: Releasing Unwanted Spirits from Your Energy Body.* Charlottesville, N.C.: Hampton Roads.

Bardeau, Fabrice. 1993. *Die Apotheke Gottes.* Translated into German by Karl H. Kosmehl. Frankfurt am Main/Berlin: Ullstein.

Bartens, Werner. 2006. *Lexikon der Medizinirrtümer.* Frankfurt am Main: Eichborn.

Bäumler, Siegfried. 2007. *Heilpflanzen Praxis heute.* Munich and Jena: Urban & Fischer.

Beyer, Rolf. 1996. *Die andere Offenbarung.* Wiesbaden: Fourier.

Bichmann, Wolfgang. 1995. "Gesundheitssysteme im internationalen Kontext: Der Blick nach draußen." In *Ritual und Heilung,* edited by Beatrix Pfleiderer, Katarina Greifeld, and Wolfgang Bichmann. Berlin: Reimer.

Bigelsen, Harvey. 2011. *Doctors Are More Harmful Than Germs.* Berkeley, Calif.: North Atlantic.

Blech, Jörg. 2005. *Fragwürdige Therapien und wie Sie sich davor schützen können.* Frankfurt am Main: Fischer.

Blüchel, Kurt G. 2003. *Heilen verboten, töten erlaubt.* Munich: Bertelsmann.

Blumert, Michael, and Jialiu Liu. 2012. *Jiaogulan: China's "Immortality" Herb.* Miramonte, Calif.: Torchlight.

Bock, Hieronymus. 1539. *New Kreüterbuch.* Strassburg: Rihel.

Böttiger, Helmut. 2008. *Klimawandel.* Petersberg: Imhof.

Brunfels, Otto. 1532. *Contrafayt Kreüterbuch nach rechter vollkommener art, und Beschreibungen der Alten besst-beruempten aerzt, vormals in Teütscher sprach, der masszen nye gesehen, noch im Truck auszgangen.* Strassburg: Schott.

Brunschwig [Brunschwygk], Hieronymus. 1500. *Liber de arte distillandi, de simplicibus.* Strassburg: Grüninger.

Buhner, Stephen Harrod. 2002. The Lost Language of Plants. White River Junction, Vt.: Chelsea Green.

———. 2004. The Secret Teachings of Plants. Rochester, Vt.: Bear & Company.

Bühring, Ursel. 2005. *Praxis-Lehrbuch der modernen Pflanzenheilkunde.* Stuttgart: Sonntag.

———. 2007. *Alles über Heilpflanzen.* Stuttgart: Ulmer.

Burton, Robert. 1628. *The Anatomie of Melancholy: What it Is, with All the Kinds, Causes, Symptomes, Prognostickes, and Seuerall Cures of it.* Oxford: Cripps.

Cannon, Walter B. 1965. "Voodoo Death." In *Reader in Comparative Religion: An Anthropological Approach,* edited by William A. Lessa and Evon Z. Vogt. New York: Harper & Row. [Reprint from *American Anthropologist* 44.2 (1942): 169–81.]

Carl, Helmut. 1957. *Die deutschen Pflanzen– und Tiernamen: Deutung und sprachliche Ordnung.* Wiebelsheim, Germany: Quelle & Meyer.

Chopra, Deepak. 2001. *Healing the Heart.* London: Rider.

Coleman, Vernon. 2006. *How to Stop Your Doctor Killing You.* Batu Caves, Selangor: Masterpiece.

Culpeper, Nicholas. 1999 [1653]. *The Complete Herbal.* Delhi: Sri Satguru.

Dash, Bhagwan. 1995. *Ayurvedic Cures for Common Diseases.* Delhi: Hind.

Davidson, Michael W., ed. 1992. The Field Guide to the Wild Flowers of Britain. London: Berkeley Square House.

Dinzelbacher, Peter. 1995. *Heilige oder Hexen?* Zurich: Artemis.

Engels, Friedrich. 2009 [1845]. *The Condition of the Working Class in England.* London: Penguin Classics.

Erichsen-Brown, Charlotte. 1979. *Medicinal and Other Uses of North American Plants.* New York: Dover.

Frazer, James G. 1951. *The Golden Bough.* New York: Macmillan.

Friedl, Reinhard. 2019. *Der Takt des Lebens.* Munich: Random House.

Friedman, Meyer, and Ray H. Rosenman. 1974. *Type A Behavior and Your Heart.* New York: Knopf.

Frohn, Birgit. 2001. *Klostermedizin*. Munich: DTV.

Früh, Sigrid, ed. 1996. *Märchenreise durch Deutschland*. Frankfurt am Main: Fischer.

Fuchs, Leonhart. 1543. *New Kreüterbuch*. Basel: Isingrin.

Fulder, Stephen. 1985. *Tao der Medizin*. Basel: Sphinx.

Gallwitz, Esther. 1992. *Kleiner Kräutergarten*. Frankfurt am Main and Leipzig: Insel.

Garrett, Laurie. 2011. *Betrayal of Trust*. New York: Hachette.

Geesing, Hermann. 2003. *Herz-Fit*. Munich: Herbig.

Goethe, Johann Wolfgang. 1948. *Gesamtausgabe*. Zurich: Beutler.

———. 1998. *Poems of the West and East: West-Eastern Divan / West-Östlicher Divan: Bi-Lingual Edition of the Complete Poems*. Translated by John Whaley. Bern: Lang.

Grabner-Haider, Anton, and Helma Marx. 2005. *Das Buch der Mythen aller Zeiten und Völker*. Wiesbaden: Marix.

Grieve, Maude. 1981. *A Modern Herbal*. New York: Dover.

Griffith, Ralph T. H., trans. 1889–1892. *The Hymns of the Rigveda*. Second edition. 4 vols. Benares: Lazarus.

Grimm, Jacob. 2003 [1875–1878]. *Deutsche Mythologie*. Wiesbaden: Fourier.

Grimm, Jacob, and Wilhelm Grimm. 1877. *Deutsches Wörterbuch*. 16 vols. Leipzig: Hirzel.

———. 1922. *Kinder- und Hausmärchen*. 3 vols. Marburg: Elwert.

———. 2004. *Selected Tales*. Translated by David Luke. London: Penguin.

Habinger-Tuczay, Christa. 1992. *Magie und Magier im Mittelalter*. Munich: Diederichs.

Hageneder, Fred. 2001. *The Heritage of Trees*. Edinburgh: Floris.

Harris, Marvin. 2005. *Wohlgeschmack und Widerwillen*. Stuttgart: Klett.

Hasenfratz, Hans-Peter. 2011. *Barbarian Rites: The Spiritual World of the Vikings and the Germanic Tribes*. Translated and edited by Michael Moynihan. Rochester, Vt.: Inner Traditions.

Hegi, Gustav. 1906–1931. *Illustrierte Flora von Mittel-Europa*. 7 vols. Vienna: Pichler.

Heidelberger, Michael, and Sigrun Thiessen. 1981. *Natur und Erfahrung*. Reinbek bei Hamburg: Rowohlt.

Heine, Heinrich. *The Poems of Heine*. Translated by Edgar Alfred Bowring. London: Bell and Sons, 1908.

Heinrich, Michael. 2001. *Ethnopharmazie und Ethnobotanik*. Stuttgart: Wissenschaftliche Verlagsgesellschaft.

Heise, Thomas. 1996. *Chinas Medizin bei uns*. Berlin: VWB.

Hempen, Carl-Hermann, and Toni Fischer. 2007. *Leitfaden Chinesische Phythotherapie*. Munich and Jena: Urban & Fischer.

Herrera, Emilio, and Maria Pilar Ramos. 2008. "Long-Term Effects of Trans Fatty Acid Intake during Pregnancy and Lactation: Does It Have Deleterious Consequences?" *Future Lipidology* 3 (5): 489–94.

Hildegard of Bingen. 1957. *Heilkunde*. Salzburg: Müller.

———. 1998. *Physica*. Translated by Priscilla Throop. Rochester, Vt.: Healing Arts Press.

———. 2007. *Liber simplices medicinae (Das Buch der Pflanzen)*. Salzburg: Müller.

———. 2010. *Physica: Liber subtilitatum diversarum naturarum creaturarum*, vol. 1. Edited by Reiner Hildebrandt and Thomas Gloning. Berlin: De Gruyter.

Hiller, Karl, and Matthias F. Melzig. 2003. *Lexikon der Arzneipflanzen und Drogen*. Heidelberg and Berlin: Spektrum.

Hoerner, Wilhelm. 1993. *Zeit und Rhythmus: Die Ordnungsgesetze der Erde und des Menschen*. Stuttgart: Urachhaus.

Horace. *The Odes, Epodes, Satires, and Epistles*. Translated by Ben Johnson et al. London and New York: Warne, 1889.

Hovorka, Oskar von, and Adolf Kronfeld. 1909. *Vergleichende Volksmedizin: Eine Darstellung volksmedizinischer Sitten und Gebräuche*. 2 vols. Stuttgart: Strecker & Schröder.

Hufeland, Christoph Wilhelm. 1799. *Die Kunst das menschliche Leben zu verlängern* [The art of lengthening human life]. Jena: Akademische Buchhandlung.

Hultkrantz, Åke. 1992. *Shamanic Healing and Ritual Drama*. New York: Crossroad.

Huxley, Francis. 1976. *The Way of the Sacred*. New York: Dell.

Kaden, Marion. 2007. "Dorniger Geselle mit Herz." *Natürlich* (March issue).

Kalweit, Holger. 2006. *Das Totenbuch der Kelten*. Düsseldorf: Albatros.

Keller, Erich. 1999. *Aromatherapy Handbook for Beauty, Hair, and Skin Care*. Rochester, Vt.: Healing Arts Press.

Knappert, Jan. 1994. *Lexikon der indischen Mythologie*. Munich: Heyne.

Kneipp, Sebastian. 1894. *Meine Wasserkur*. Kempten: Kösel.

Köbl, Konrad. 1993. *Köbl's Kräuterfiebel*. Munich: Köbl.

Konrad von Megenberg. 1989. *Buch der Natur*. Translated by Gerhard E. Sollbach. Dortmund: Harenberg-Edition.

Konz, Franz. 2000. *Der große Gesundheits-Konz*. Munich: Universitas.

Kumar, K. Parvathi. 2003. *Shirdi Sai Sayings*. Chennai: Dhanishta.

Künzle, Johann. 1945. *Das große Kräuterbuch*. Olten: Walter.

———. 2008 [1911]. *Chrut und Uchrut*. Baden: AT Verlag.

Lazarou, J., et al. 1998. "Incidence of Adverse Drug Reactions in Hospitalized Patients." *Journal of the American Medical Association* 279 (15): 1200–205.

Legros, Waltraud. 2003. *Was die Wörter erzählen*. Munich: DTV.

Lipp, Frank J. *Herbalism*. 1996. Boston: Little, Brown.

Lonicerus, Adamus. 1679. *Kreuterbuch*. Frankfurt: Wagner.

Ludvik, Catherine. 1997. *Hanumān: In the Rāmayāṇa of Vālmīki and the Rāmacaritamānasa of Tulasī Dāsa*. Delhi: Banarsidass.

Lurker, Manfred. 1981. *Götter und Symbole der alten Ägypter*. Munich: Goldmann.

Luther, Martin. 1898. *Sämmtliche Schriften*, vol 14. Edited by Johannes Georg Walch. St. Louis, Mo.: Concordia.

Mabey, Richard. 1993. *Das neue BLV Buch der Kräuter*. Munich: BLV.

Madaus, Gerhard. 1979 [1938]. *Lehrbuch der biologischen Heilmittel*. 3 vols. Hildesheim: Olms.

Mangan, James Clarence. 1870. *Poems*. New York: Haverty.

Marzell, Heinrich. 2002 [1938]. *Geschichte und Volkskunde der deutschen Heilpflanzen*. St. Goar: Reichl.

———. 1943–1979. *Wörterbuch der deutschen Pflanzennamen*. 5 vols. Leipzig: Hirzel.

Mattioli, Pietro Andrea. 1563. Translated into German by Georg Handsch. *New Kreüterbuch*. Prague and Venice: Melantrich and Valgrisi.

Mauch, Walter. 2007. *Die Bombe in der Achselhöhle*. Munich: Bettendorf.

Maxen, Andreas von, Gabi Hoffbauer, and Andreas Heeke. 2005. *Kursbuch: Medikamente und Wirkstoffe*. Augsburg: Weltbild.

McIntyre, Anne. 2019. *The Complete Herbal Tutor*. London: Aeon.

McLuhan, T. C. 1972. *Touch the Earth*. New York: Outerbridge & Dienstfrey.

McTagggart, Lynne. 2000. *What Doctors Don't Tell You: The Truth About the Dangers of Modern Medicine*. London: Thorsons.

Merchant, Carolyn. 1990. *The Death of Nature: Women, Ecology, and the Scientific Revolution*. San Francisco: HarperOne.

Minker, Margaret. 1992. *Wörterbuch der Medizin*. Niedernhausen: Falken.

Müller, Ingo Wilhelm. 1993. *Humoralmedizin*. Heidelberg: Haug.

Müller, Irmgard. 1982. "Einführung des Kaffees in Europa." In *Rausch und Realität: Drogen im Kulturvergleich,* edited by Gisela Völger and Karin von Welck. 3 vols. Reinbek bei Hamburg: Rowohlt.

———. 1993. *Die pflanzlichen Heilmittel bei Hildegard von Bingen.* Freiburg im Breisgau: Herder Spektrum.

Nager, Frank. 1992. *Der heilkundige Dichter: Goethe und die Medizin.* Düsseldorf and Zurich: Artemis & Winkler.

Nettle, Daniel, and Suzanne Romaine. 2000. *Vanishing Voices.* New York: Oxford University Press.

Neuwinger, Hans Dieter. 1998. *Afrikanische Arzneipflanzen und Jagdgifte: Chemie, Pharmakologie, Toxikologie.* Stuttgart: WVG.

Novalis. 1980. *Im Einverständnis mit dem Geheimnis.* Freiburg im Breisgau: Herder.

Orth, Gerhard. 1996. *Unheilbare Krankheiten.* Ritterhude: Waldthausen.

Ots, Thomas. 1990. *Medizin und Heilung in China.* Berlin: Reimer.

Pahlow, Mannfried. 1979. *Das große Buch der Heilpflanzen: Gesund durch die Heilkräfte der Natur.* Munich: Gräfe und Unzer.

Patnaik, Naveen. 1993. *The Garden of Life.* New York: Doubleday.

Paullini, Christian Franz. 1734. *Neu-Vermehrte, Heylsame Dreckapotheke.* Frankfurt: Koch.

Pearsall, Paul. 1999. *The Heart's Code.* New York: Harmony.

Pearsall, Paul, Gary E. R. Schwartz, and Linda G. S. Russek. 2002. "Changes in Heart Transplant Recipients that Parallel the Personalities of their Donors." *Journal of Near-Death Studies* 20.3: 191–206.

Pelikan, Wilhelm. 1975. *Heilpflanzenkunde.* 3 vols. Dornach: Philosophisch-Anthroposophischer Verlag.

Pelletier, Kenneth R., ed. 2007. *New Medicine.* London: DK.

Perger, K. Ritter von. 1864. *Deutsche Pflanzensagen.* Stuttgart and Oehringen: Schaber.

Petry, Rolf-Jürgen, and Hans Schaefer. 2007. *Die Lösung des Herzinfarkt-Problems durch Strophanthin.* Bremen: Florilegium.

Pfeifer, Wolfgang, ed. 1995. *Etymologisches Wörterbuch des Deutschen.* Munich: DTV.

Pfleiderer, Beatrix, Katarina Greifeld, and Wolfgang Bichmann. 1995. *Ritual und Heilung.* Berlin: Reimer.

Phaneuf, Holly. 2005. *Herbs Demystified.* New York: Marlowe.

Pliny. 1945. *Natural History,* vol. IV. Edited with a translation by H. Rackham. Cambridge, Mass.: Harvard University Press.

———. 1966. *Natural History,* vol. VII. Edited with a translation by W. H. S. Jones. Cambridge, Mass.: Harvard University Press.

Pollmer, Udo, and Susanne Warmuth. 2003. *Lexikon der populären Ernährungsirrtümer.* Augsburg: Weltbild.

Pörksen, Gunhild, ed. and trans. 1988. *Paracelsus: Vom eigenen Vermögen der Natur. Frühe Schriften zur Heilmittellehre.* Frankfurt am Main: Fischer.

Porter, Roy. 1999. *The Greatest Benefit to Mankind: A Medical History of Humanity.* New York: Norton.

Rätsch, Christian. 2002. "Zaubersprüche als Therapie—zur Ethnomedizin der Lakandonen im mexikanischen Regenwald." In *Handbuch der Ethnotherapien / Handbook of Ethnotherapies,* edited by Christine E. Gottschalk-Batschkus and Joy C. Green. Munich: Ethnomed.

Reinhard, Jürg, and A. Baumann. 1992. *Unerhörtes aus der Medizin.* Bern: Hallwag.

Reinhard, Jürg. 2008. *Sanfte Heilpraxis mit selbstgemachten Medikamenten.* Baden: AT Verlag.

Rippe, Olaf, Margret Madejsky, Max Amann, Patricia Ochsner, and Christian Rätsch. 2001. *Paracelsusmedizin: Altes Wissen in der Heilkunde von heute. Philosophie, Astrologie, Alchimie, Therapiekonzepte.* Aarau: AT Verlag.

Rippe, Olaf, and Margret Madejsky. 2006. *Die Kräuterkunde des Paracelsus.* Baden and Munich: AT Verlag.

Rippe, Olaf. 2005. "Mut und Willensstärke durch Kräuter." In *Naturheilpraxis Spezial: Traditionelle Abendländische Medizin.* Munich: Pflaum.

Röhrich, Lutz. 2001. *Lexikon der sprichwörtlichen Redensarten,* vol. 2. Freiburg: Herder.

Rosenman, Ray H., Meyer Friedman, et al. 1964. "A Predictive Study of Coronary Heart Disease: The Western Collaborative Group Study." *Journal of the American Medical Association* 189.1: 15–26.

Sahlins, Marshall. 1972. *Stone Age Economics.* New York: Aldine.

Scheffer, Mechthild and Wolf-Dieter Storl. 2007. *Die Seelenpflanzen des Edward Bach.* Kreuzlingen and Munich: Hugendubel.

Schiller, Friedrich. 1875. *Die Piccolomini.* Edited by James Morgan Hart. New York: Putnam's.

Schiller, Reinhard. 1991. *Hildegard Pflanzenapotheke.* Augsburg: Pattloch.

Schmertzing, Georg. 2002. *Kraftfeld Herz.* Güllesheim: Silberschnur.

Schmidsberger, Peter. 1990. *Heilpflanzen.* Bindlach: Gondrom.

Schmidt, Heinrich, and Georgi Schischkof. 1978. *Philosophisches Wörterbuch.* Stuttgart: Kröner.

Schnurrer, J. U., and J. C. Fröhlich. 2003. "Zur Häufigkeit und Vermeidbarkeit von tödlichen unerwünschten Arzneimittelwirkungen." *Die Innere Medizin* 44.7: 889–95.

Schöffer, Peter. *Gart der Gesundheit.* 1485. Mainz.

Schönfelder, Peter, and Ingrid Schönfelder. 2004. *Das neue Handbuch der Heilpflanzen*. Stuttgart: Franckh-Kosmos.

Schrödter, Willy. 1997. *Pflanzen-Geheimnisse*. St. Goar: Reichl.

Schwartz, Gary E. R., and Linda G. S. Russek. 1999. *The Living Energy Universe*. Charlottesville, Va.: Hampton Roads.

Schwemmer, Ulrike. 2000. *Medizin im neuen Jahrtausend*. Vienna and Munich: Deutike.

Sheldrake, Rupert. 1994. *The Rebirth of Nature: The Greening of Science and God*. Rochester, Vt.: Park Street.

Simonis, Werner Christian. 1970. *Der rote Fingerhut*. Dornach: Philosophisch-Anthroposophischer Verlag am Goetheanum.

Steiner, Rudolf. 1961. *Geisteswissenschaft und Medizin*. Dornach: Rudolf Steiner Nachlassverwaltung, 1961. [English edition: *Introducing Anthroposophical Medicine*, translated by Catherine E. Creeger. Hudson, N.Y.: Anthroposophic Press, 1999.]

Stoffler, Hans-Dieter. 2002. *Kräuter aus dem Klostergarten*. Stuttgart: Thorbecke.

Storl, Wolf-Dieter. 2000. *Pflanzen der Kelten*. Aarau: AT Verlag.

———. 2003. *Ich bin ein Teil des Waldes*. Stuttgart: Kosmos.

———. 2004a. *Shiva: The Wild God of Power and Ecstasy*. Rochester, Vt.: Inner Traditions.

———. 2004b. *Von Heilkräutern und Pflanzengottheiten*. Bielefeld: Kamphausen.

———. 2005a. *Naturrituale*. Baden and Munich: AT Verlag.

———. 2005b. "Würmlein klein, ohne Haut und Bein—schamanische und ethnobotanische Aspekte der indigenen Heilkunde Nordeuropas." In *Der große Lebenskreis: Ethnotherapien im Kreislauf von Vergehen, Sein und Werden*, edited by Christine E. Gottschalk-Batschkus and Joy C. Green. Munich: Ethnomed.

———. 2006a. *Streifzüge am Rande Midgards*. Burgrain: KOHA.

———. 2006b. *Kräuterkunde*. Bielefeld: Aurum in J. Kamphausen.

———. 2008. "Vorwort" in *Meine Heilpflanzen* by Maria Treben. Steyr: Ennsthaler.

———. 2012. The Herbal Lore of Wise Women and Wortcunners: *The Healing Power of Medicinal Plants*. Berkeley, Calif.: North Atlantic.

———. 2013. *Culture and Horticulture: The Classic Guide to Biodynamic and Organic Gardening*. Berkeley, Calif.: North Atlantic.

———. 2018a. *Bear: Myth—Animal—Icon*. Berkeley, Calif.: North Atlantic.

———. 2018b. "Indo-European Healing Lore." *TYR* 5: 172–222.

Sudhoff, Karl, ed. 1922–1933. *Theophrast von Hohenheim: Medizinische, naturwissenschaftliche und philosophische Schriften des Paracelsus.* 14 vols. Munich and Berlin: Verlag Oldenbourg.

Sylvia, Claire, with William Novak. 1997. *A Change of Heart.* Boston: Little, Brown and Company.

Tabernaemontanus, Jacobus Theodorus. 1588–1591. *Neuw Kreuterbuch.* Frankfurt: Bassaeus.

Tietze, Henry G. 1987. *Entschlüsselte Organsprache.* Munich: Knaur.

Treben, Maria. 2017. *Health Through God's Pharmacy: Advice and Proven Cures with Medicinal Herbs.* Steyr: Ennsthaler.

Vries, Herman de. 2000. "Heilige Bäume, Bilsenkraut und Bildzeitung." In *Rituale des Heilens: Ethnomedizin, Naturerkenntnis und Heilkraft,* edited by Franz-Theo Gottwald and Christian Rätsch. Aarau: AT Verlag.

Waldenberger, Ferdinand R. 2003. *Handbuch für Herzbesitzer.* Wien: Ueberreuter.

Walker, Barbara G. 2003. *Das geheime Wissen der Frauen.* Engerda: Arun.

Watts, Alan. 1975. *Tao: The Watercourse Way.* New York: Pantheon.

WebMD. 2020. "Heart Failure and Heart Transplants." Medically reviewed by James Beckerman, M.D, FACC on July 15, 2020.

Weil, Andrew. 1983. *Health and Healing: Understanding Conventional and Alternative Medicine.* Boston: Houghton Mifflin Harcourt.

———. 2000. *Spontaneous Healing: How to Discover and Embrace Your Body's Natural Ability to Maintain and Heal Itself.* New York: Ballantine.

Weiss, Rudolf Fritz. 2001. *Weiss's Herbal Medicine.* New York: Thieme.

Weiss, Rudolf Fritz, and Volker Fintelmann. 2002. *Lehrbuch der Phythotherapie.* Stuttgart: Hippokrates.

Willett, W. C., M. J. Stampfer, J. E. Manson, G. A. Colditz, F. E. Speizer, B. A. Rosner, C. H. Hennekens, et al. 1993. "Intake of Trans Fatty Acids and Risk of Coronary Heart Disease among Women." *The Lancet* 341 (8845): P581–85.

Willett, W. C., M. J. Stampfer, J. E. Manson, G. A. Colditz, B. A. Rosner, F. E. Speizer, and C. H. Hennekens. 1996. "Coffee Consumption and Coronary Heart Disease in Women: A Ten-Year Follow-Up." JAMA 275 (6):458-62.

Wolters, Bruno. 1999. "Die ältesten Heilpflanzen." *Deutsche Apotheker Zeitung* 39 (Sept. 30).

Zacharias, Irmgard. 1982. *Die Sprache der Blumen.* Rosenheim: Rosenheimer.

Zerling, Clemens. 2007. *Lexikon der Pflanzensymbolik.* Baden and Munich: AT Verlag.

Zoller, Andrea, and Hellmuth Nordwig. 1997. *Heilpflanzen der Ayurvedischen Medizin.* Heidelberg: Haug.

Photo Credits

Photographs by Frank Brunke: alpine lovage (p. 146), bear leek (pp. 148), bear wort (pp. 150, 151), blue fragrant violet (p. 152), bog star (p. 157), borage seeds (p. 158), hedge woundwort (p. 166), key flower (pp. xiv, 168), lemon balm (pp. 170, 172), linden tree (p. 175), milk thistle seeds (p. 180), mullein (p. 182), oregano (pp. vi, 184, 185) raspberry (p. 187), rose (p. 188), rosemary (p. 193), speedwell (p. 194), storksbill (p. 200), strawberry (p. 203), valerian (p. 204), vervain (p. 209), woodruff (p. 212), green hellebore (p. 223), black hellebore (p. 223), lily of the valley (p. 229), spring pheasant's eye (p. 237), wallflower (pp. 239, 240), garlic (p. 241), hawthorn (p. 242), mistletoe (pp. 246, 247), motherwort (p. 251), mountain arnica (pp. 254, 255), periwinkle (p. 261), Scotch broom (p. 262)

Photographs by Ingrid Lisa Storl: borage (p. 158), chamomile (p. 163), daisy (p. 164), linden leaf (p. 176), milk thistle blossom (p. 179), St. John's wort (p. 196), and foxglove (p. 217)

Photographs from Wikimedia Commons: *CC BY-SA 2.0*—Indian snakeroot (p. 273) by Dinesh Valke. *CC BY-SA 3.0*—queen of the night (p. 235) by Sadambio, arjun tree (p. 264) by Linél, coffee (p. 267) by H. Zell, jiaogulan (p. 276) by Doronenko, poison rope (p. 278) by JMK. *CC BY 3.0 US*—yellow oleander (p. 282) by Forest & Kim Starr. *CC BY-SA 4.0*—oleander (p. 234) by Jim Evans, squill (p. 238) by Zeynel Cebeci, ginkgo (p. 270) by Krzysztof Ziarnek, Kenraiz

INDEX

ABOUT THE AUTHOR

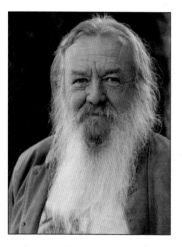

WOLF D. STORL, Ph.D., born in 1942 in Saxony, Germany, is a cultural anthropologist and ethnobotanist. At the age of eleven he immigrated with his parents to the United States, where he spent most of his free time in the forest wilderness of Ohio.

When he was nineteen he enrolled as a botany student at Ohio State University, but bored with dry laboratory work, he soon switched to anthropology. After graduation, he became an assistant then full-time lecturer in sociology and anthropology at Kent State University. In 1974 he received his doctorate in ethnology (magna cum laude) as a Fulbright scholar from Bern, Switzerland. This was followed by teaching positions at the Institute for International Studies (Vienna), Rogue College (Oregon), and the Seminary pour la Formation de Socio-Therapeutes (Geneva). He was also a guest lecturer for cultural ecology at the University of Bern, a visiting scholar at the Benares Hindu University, and an adjunct professor at Sheridan College (Wyoming).

Numerous trips, including ethnographic and ethnobotanical field research, shaped Storl's thinking. His experiences—with a spiritualist settlement in Ohio; a Camphill community south of Geneva,

Switzerland, among biodynamic farmers in the Emmental; and with Cheyenne medicine men and Shiva sadhus in India and Nepal—are reflected in his numerous publications.

Wild, primordial nature has always been his inspiration and has formed his philosophy of life. For Storl, plants are not only botanical objects—they have a cultural, linguistic, medicinal, and mythological identity through their interrelationship with humans.

The scholar, speaker, and author lives with his family in the Allgäu region of southern Germany.

Visit his website at **www.storl.de/english-books-by-wolf-d-storl**.

OTHER BOOKS BY WOLF D. STORL, PH.D.

Far Out in America: A German Ethnobotanist's Wild Roots in the Psychedelic Sixties, (Arcana Europa Media: Wild Lives, 2021)

On the Banks of the Ganges: A Young Anthropologist Couple's Adventures in India (Outskirts, 2019)

Bear: Myth, Animal, Icon (North Atlantic, 2018)

The Untold History of Healing: Plant Lore and Medicinal Magic from the Stone Age to Present (North Atlantic, 2017)

A Curious History of Vegetables: Aphrodisiacal and Healing Properties, Folk Tales, Garden Tips, and Recipes (North Atlantic, 2016)

Culture and Horticulture: The Classic Guide to Biodynamic and Organic Gardening, revised edition (North Atlantic, 2013)

The Herbal Lore of Wise Women and Wortcunners: The Healing Power of Medicinal Plants (North Atlantic, 2012)

Healing Lyme Disease Naturally: History, Analysis, and Treatments (North Atlantic, 2010)

Shiva: The Wild God of Power and Ecstasy (Inner Traditions, 2004)

Witchcraft Medicine: Healing Arts, Shamanic Practices, and Forbidden Plants, with Claudia Müller-Ebeling and Christian Rätsch (Inner Traditions, 2003)

BOOKS OF RELATED INTEREST

Witchcraft Medicine
Healing Arts, Shamanic Practices, and Forbidden Plants
*by Claudia Müller-Ebeling, Christian Rätsch,
and Wolf-Dieter Storl, Ph.D.*

Bach Flower Therapy
Theory and Practice
by Mechthild Scheffer

The Herbal Handbook
A User's Guide to Medical Herbalism
by David Hoffmann, FNIMH, AHG

Medical Herbalism
The Science and Practice of Herbal Medicine
by David Hoffmann, FNIMH, AHG

Adaptogens
Herbs for Strength, Stamina, and Stress Relief
*by David Winston, RH(AHG)
with Steven Maimes*

Natural Remedies for Mental and Emotional Health
Holistic Methods and Techniques for a Happy and Healthy Mind
*by Brigitte Mars, A.H.G. and Chrystle Fiedler
Foreword by Rosemary Gladstar*

Holistic Medicine and the Extracellular Matrix
The Science of Healing at the Cellular Level
*by Matthew Wood
Foreword by Stephen Harrod Buhner*

Natural Antibiotics and Antivirals
18 Infection-Fighting Herbs and Essential Oils
by Christopher Vasey, N.D.

INNER TRADITIONS • BEAR & COMPANY
P.O. Box 388 • Rochester, VT 05767
1-800-246-8648 • www.InnerTraditions.com

Or contact your local bookseller